MAMMA CALLED
THE DOCTOR

By: Antoinette Romana

iUniverse, Inc.
New York Bloomington

Mamma Called the Doctor

This book is a work of non-fiction. As per the author all the information contained in this book is a true account of the authors recollection and in some cases, names of people and places have been altered to protect their privacy.

iUniverse books may be ordered through booksellers or by contacting:

iUniverse
1663 Liberty Drive
Bloomington, IN 47403
www.iuniverse.com
1-800-Authors (1-800-288-4677)

Because of the dynamic nature of the Internet, any Web addresses or links contained in this book may have changed since publication and may no longer be valid. The views expressed in this work are solely those of the author and do not necessarily reflect the views of the publisher, and the publisher hereby disclaims any responsibility for them.

ISBN: 978-1-4401-2544-7 (pbk)
ISBN: 978-1-4401-2505-8 (cloth)
ISBN: 978-1-4401-0260-8 (ebk)

Printed in the United States of America

iUniverse rev. date: 2/11/2009

My story is dedicated to all mothers.

Every day we make simple decisions to keep our children safe.

We try to protect our children from hurting themselves. We try to teach them right from wrong. We even try to teach them about strangers. Some days our tasks are simple and make sense. Other days are harder and we pray our decisions are for the best.

At the end of the day we thank God for keeping our children safe and we ask God to forgive us for wrong choices.

- 1 -
Preface

Every day I kiss my children good morning and every day I look up into the sky to say good morning to my fourth child in heaven. I sit at the kitchen table with paper and pen in hand. This is my way of communicating to my loved ones who live in heaven. I have no idea why I have a need to air all my dirty laundry on paper. I guess that when I write it down it reminds me that this is my life.

I have discovered that bad things really do happen to good people. I know that I am a good person. I try at least to do right by my husband and children. Everyone else is secondary in my life and my concerns do not rely on their happiness. I would have done anything to ensure my son Luca's well being. I could not guarantee him a good future here on earth. Hell I could not even guarantee that I would live long enough to take care of him. It has taken me a long time to accept my choices and appreciate the strength Angelo and I needed to offer our child back to God.

Everyone has moved on over the years and I still need to write down all of my thoughts. I guess it keeps my story alive when I see it in black and white. I sometimes wonder how many women have had to face a similar situation and how many of them have followed in my footsteps. I also wonder how many people would throw a brick at my front door in disgust if they heard my story. Most of all I wonder how many families are raising special needs children and whether they would understand my decision or secretly wish they had done the same. Four years later I am still not sure whether I made the best decision, but I do know I made the right decision for our child. It is what it is. No one on this earth is without sin. No one on this earth has the right to cast the first stone. I have taken on the most difficult job in the world. I am trying my best to raise strong and happy children. I did not know if I was able to do that for Luca.

- 2 -
A Wedding

February 27, 2004, my heart jumped into my throat when I heard her voice on the other end of the line. In that split moment I thought, "No way. She just forgot to ask me to sign some papers." My heart pounded, and I heard the words "I'm sorry Antoinette the test proved positive for Downs Syndrome." I held the phone tightly to my ear hoping that if I did not say anything the test would change to negative, but it did not happen. I had been standing over the sink washing dishes with no worries other than the usual concerns. I had been thinking that I needed to find a moment to pay a few bills and get the laundry done. I had even wondered what to cook for dinner just before I received my life changing call.

She went on to say, "You need to speak to Angelo, you both have a few important decisions to make." I saw myself spinning around and around; I could feel my legs beginning to shake, and I felt weak. All I could say was, "I'll have to call you back."

I slid down to the ground and cried like a baby. I couldn't catch my breath and I could feel my throat dry up and swell. My face became hotter and hotter, and my hands trembled. I wrapped my arms around my belly and looking down the only thought in my mind was, "what do I do, what in God's name do I do?"

The first person that came to my mind was Angelo, my husband, and I remembered the first evening we met. I was invited to a friend's wedding along with a few girlfriends. I had just turned 30 a couple of months before and I was beginning to feel like an old lonely maid. I made a conscious effort to look my best: wore my navy blue dress, with an open back and v-neck line that showed just a hint of cleavage. The dress embraced every curve of my shapely body and reaching just above my knee. I wore the black sling back heels and had to walk on my toes to support myself. I had gone to the hairdresser earlier that day to straighten my bleached blond hair. I was careful with every detail of my makeup, enhancing my lashes and adding a subtle pink to my cheeks. I wore my favorite lipstick, "devil red." I wanted to have the reddest, most luscious lips that any man would kill for, for just one kiss.

I felt pretty that day and the possibility of meeting an eligible bachelor at the wedding was on my mind. As I began to walk through the receiving line, I did not pay much attention to the bridesmaids but glanced towards the ushers. I recognized some as the bride's family members and knew a few of them were married. Half way down the receiving line, someone caught my eye and I wondered who he was. As I leaned over to kiss the bride on her cheek, we exchanged a few words but, all the while, my true focus was on the handsome usher.

He was tall and slender and his shoulders were those of a football player. He had gorgeous hazel eyes and curly black long hair. He was laughing and toasting everyone with zambucca shots. I stared at him just long enough to catch his eye, and smiled; I did not want to appear too anxious, so I did not show my teeth. He continued to look at me, and after raising a shot glass in my direction as he leaned his head back and let the clear drink enter his mouth. I turned to walk away, giggling. "God I'm good." I thought.

I was seated at a table with friends I had known for 15 years. We took turns pointing out handsome men but then we noticed their wives. The conversation was light and jolly. After dinner when the D.J. loudly announced the first dance, I had a feeling it was going to be a long night of drinking wine and sitting for me; but a gentleman had approached my table and as I looked up, I saw that it was the dark handsome usher who stood across from me. With his eyes gazing directly at me he leaned forward and placing his hands on two chairs, supporting his weight. I stared back, wondering, "Who is he going to ask to dance?"

I became excited as I waited for his first words. "I have to ask you to dance." He said. I wanted to jump out of my seat and drag him off to the dance floor. Instead, I answered sarcastically, "You don't have to do anything!" At the same time I could hear a voice in my mind saying, "You idiot, don't challenge him. No wonder you're not married." I smiled nervously, expecting him to stand tall and walk away; but he stood tall and said, "Okay I would like to ask you to dance." I wanted to make the cross but silently whispered "Thank God", and followed him to the dance floor.

It was a slow song and he placed his right hand on my back, touching my bare skin, placing his left hand over my right and drawing it to his chest. He then gently pulled me toward his body, and I could smell the sweetness of his cologne; we both smiled. I was enjoying the moment, thinking, "He is very tall, even with my heels on." He wasted no time asking questions, "What part of Italy are you from?" I smiled and said proudly, "I'm Sicilian and you?" "I'm from the city of Rome." he answered, and asked me if I spoke Italian fluently. " I speak Sicilian fluently." I could tell by his smile that he was pleased and he pulled me closer for the rest of the dance.

We paid attention to no one but each other for the rest of the evening. We rocked and rolled, twisting our hips from side to side. We disco danced, and I laughed when I saw Angelo wave his arms every which way, and of course we attempted Italian dances like the tarantellas.

In between dances, we went to the bar to quench our thirst, and took a couple of minutes to go outside so that Angelo could smoke a cigarette. As he lit his cigarette he asked me where I worked. I answered that I am a data entry clerk for a transport company and have been at the same company for nine years. He said he worked for a large food distributor, and I discovered that he worked five minutes away from my office. As our conversation proceeded, I could not wait any longer and asked, "How old are you?" He started to smile and said, "Does it matter?" "No, I'm just curious." I answered. But I thought "you're damn right it matters; I'm 30 years old and my clock is ticking, buddy." He leaned into me and said, "I'm 27." He did not take his eyes off me, and placed his cigarette in his lips waiting for my reaction. "Oh, I'm 30." I said. He quickly changed the topic and we continued talking.

The evening came to an end. The bride and groom had given their speeches, and the dim lights that gave the room a romantic ambiance, were now bright. I realized I had not been back to my table since the first dance, and knew that my friends were now, not only gathering their belongings, but itching to ask me a million questions.

Although I did not want the evening to end, I said good bye to Angelo. "I had a wonderful evening. Thank you for being a great dance partner and for saving me from a dreadful evening." I said, and began to walk away hoping he would follow. Every step took me further and further away from our heavenly evening. When I leaned forward to take my purse from my table there was a tap on my shoulder. Even though I was excited I had been dreading this moment. Do I wait for him to offer me his phone number? Do I offer him mine? Do I kiss him on the cheek or shake his hand? I decided to follow his lead, thinking, "If he just says good-bye, I will appreciate the wonderful evening and leave gracefully." but my heart was singing a different tune I really wanted his telephone number.

Angelo leaned into my shoulder and as he was about to speak, an elderly gentleman grabbed him by the shoulders and swung him around. They greeted each other with enthusiasm, and Angelo apologized for not greeting him earlier. I was completely mesmerized by Angelo's fluent Italian. The words flowed gracefully and sounded so sexy. I knew at that moment that I had to see him again.

When Angelo steered his attention back to me, he asked, "Can I see you again?" I smiled and answered, "Yes." I could hear "Halleluiah" singing loudly in my head. Angelo ran around asking everyone if they had a pen. I couldn't help but watch his desperation and giggle. I waited patiently as Angelo wrote down his phone number, cell number and work number." When he passed me a ripped cigarette box with his numbers, I laughed and said, "No pressure here!" Angelo had a big smile on his face. I stood as tall as I could, on my tippy toes, and kissed his cheek good-bye.

That night, I tossed and turned, repeating the evening's events over and over in my mind, thinking, "Could he really be the prince I have been waiting for. He seems different from the frogs I have dated." I put my hands together and prayed, "Hey God, if he is the one for me, please help our relationship move along, but if he is not my future, please do not let him pursue me. It felt good to leave my dilemma in God's hands and I finally fell asleep.

- 3 -
Angelo

My thoughts returned to the baby. I held my belly and thought, "How do I tell Angelo that his fourth child has a problem, a serious problem." I could not stop crying. My tears were for Angelo. Angelo had always said, "I'm the last male in my family to carry our name." The day our son Joseph was born, Angelo said, "Thank you for my son. Now we have a boy to continue our family name." I was happy for Angelo, and when our son Gaetano was born, I knew that our family name would grow and live on forever. Knowing that I had already given my husband two sons to carry our name was special. Three boys would have been exceptional. If it was a girl, it would have been perfect too. I couldn't stop thinking of Angelo. I knew how important it was for him to have a large family.

Angelo was born in Rome in 1968. He was the only son and the youngest of four children. When his parents came to Canada hoping for a better and prosperous life for their family, Angelo was only two months old, and his siblings were not much older. His mother had her hands full enrolling the children in school, tending to the newborn baby, and struggling with the new language. Angelo's father worked long and tedious hours to create a business and maintain the family values. They lived well, and the children did not lack a thing. They went on vacations twice a year and enjoyed adventurous outings. Angelo often told me, "My dad would call from work and tell my mom to have everyone packed up and ready to go camping for the weekend, and my mom would gather up clothes and food, and would be at the front door waiting for him when he returned."

Angelo always stressed that he wanted to have the same great memories with his own children one day.

Angelo's aunts and uncle's remained in Italy leaving Angelo's family alone in Canada, and they decided to build their own family traditions and to stay together. Angelo often said, "We have no family other than each other, and sometimes my parents miss their brothers and sisters. We call Italy often and we visit every year." But still, he felt the loneliness of being a part of a small family and he vowed to have a large family of his own.

Angelo always had great respect for his parents and appreciated his strict upbringing. While his father worked hard to support the family, Angelo had the luxury of having his mother at home. He would laugh and say, "I'm not kidding when I say that I don't know how to do any household chores." He carried the "male chauvinist" title quite proudly. As a teenager his grades were above average and according to his stories he was "quite the ladies man." He went on to university and received a bachelor's degree in Business and Italian. When he was 21, he purchased his own house with his parents help. Angelo struggled to pay the mortgage every month, but, with his full time job, he managed. He was very proud of his family values, and promised himself that one day he would follow in his parent's footsteps and raise his large family in the same way.

I sat on the floor and sobbed knowing I had a call to make, but how? I thought of calling Angelo first, but could not muster the strength to do so just yet. I reached to pick up the telephone receiver from the counter above me, and the paper with the hospitals number on it. Trying to see the phone number through my tears, I pressed each number, knowing I was getting closer to reality by calling Jane back. I heard her sweet caring voice say, "Genetics, Jane speaking. How may I help you?" Her soft voice had uttered such awful words earlier, that even her hello now felt awful. "Hi Jane it's Antoinette," my voice trembled and my hand could barely hold the receiver, it was shaking out of control. "Go ahead and make the arrangements and let me know what I need to do." I continued. "I'm going to schedule your procedure and call you back. Antoinette, I'm so sorry." She said. I knew this was not her fault, but I could not face it being my own either. What I really wanted to say was, "If you're so sorry, fix this and make it all go away." Through my crying I managed to utter the words "good-bye" and hang up.

I was crying so hard that my temples throbbed and every time a breath went in, it was as though I could not exhale. "How could this have happened to me, to us. Is it because I didn't go to church often enough; was I not grateful enough for what I had; what did we do to deserve this? " I kept thinking that there had to be a mistake, after all I had three beautiful healthy children.

- 4 -
Our Children

My son Joseph was five and in senior kindergarten. He was very smart and witty. Joseph was such a little man, and I loved talking to him. I remember when he was three years old he would always stay with me when I had a guest over or when I was on the phone. He would draw at the table, but I knew he was really listening to every word. Sometimes he repeated my words to Angelo at the most inappropriate times. I learned quickly what not to say when he was around.

When my daughter Lucy and son Gaetano were together, they would watch the same television shows or interact at a toddler's level. Joseph never really fit in with them. I would watch him wander around, or play with a toy quietly, on his own. As soon as I began to prepare dinner, Joseph would be right behind me standing no taller than the lower part of my back. "Mommy can I be your helper?" he said. I never could say no, and up he came on to the counter. I handed him a potato peeler and gave him the biggest potato, "Thank goodness you came along. I couldn't have made dinner without you." I said. When it was time to use the stove I said, "Joseph, can you please go and see what the kids are up to?" We both referred to Lucy and Gaetano as "the kids" and it made Joseph feel older and wiser than them.

Gaetano was two years old. He was a tiny child who lived and breathed dragons, aliens, and monsters. When Gaetano would put his hand to his mouth and tell me he had a secret I went down on my knees and whispered, "What's the secret?" He began with "mom, did you know that aliens live in our attic?" "Oh Gaetano, how did they get in our attic?" I asked. His eyes opened wide and he leaned closer and said, " mom, I put them there. They will be safe so no one can hurt them. I fed them bread and water, and they had their nap on the floor. You must be quiet or you will scare them." I smiled and replied, "Okay Gaetano, be very quiet when you play with your toys." Gaetano, content with his story, walked away. His imagination was so intense, I could not help but tape-record all of his stories. I know that one day he will become a writer.

Lucy was one and a half years old. She was the daughter I had always wanted. After the two boys, I prayed for a girl, and said that I would keep going until I had a daughter. Before getting pregnant for the third, time I began to read theories on how to determine the sex of a baby. I told Angelo we could only have sex on certain days in order to have a girl. Angelo would laugh and say, "I don't care how or when, as long as I get serviced." I started feeling nauseous and dizzy. I had no desire for food, and the thought of coffee made my stomach turn. I thought it might be the flu.

The doctor looked into my ears and stared down my throat. "Everything looks clear. Let's do a blood test and see if you're pregnant." He said. I started to smile. The thought of being pregnant was exciting and I was more than prepared to have anther child. The nurse came in with a large needle and a tube. I cringed. She tied a rubber band around my arm and as she slowly pushed the needle into my vein, I kept thinking, "Wow. It would be great if I was pregnant."

"What about the two week trip to Nova Scotia we planned?" Angelo asked when I returned. I looked at him and smiled, "What about it? If I'm sick, I'll take medication, and if I'm pregnant, we'll stop every once in a while so I can throw up." We both started to laugh. Gaetano was only six months old at the time, and I knew my hands were going to be very full. Two days later, I was packed and ready for our journey to Nova Scotia when someone from the doctor's office called. "I am calling to congratulate you. You are pregnant." She said. I froze for a moment, and then happy and excited said, "That's great Thank you."

I was very happy at the age of 38 with a beautiful home in the suburbs, and I was proud to call myself a stay at home mom. I had a wonderful husband who loved us and appreciated our family life. Angelo worked long hours to provide for us. Our children filled our days and brought such happiness to our home. This was our dream life; everything was just as it was supposed to be. Our lives were right on schedule, and everything was perfect.

Six weeks had passed since Lucy's birth and I needed to talk to Angelo. I had fed the children their dinner early so we would not be interrupted. I sat near Angelo at the dinner table. He lifted his cutlery and began carving his steak. It looked juicy, and I knew he was tired from work and hungry. "Angelo, I have an appointment coming up with Dr. Slater this week. I was thinking of asking him to put an IUD in." He looked at me and asked, "Why?" I watched him take another bite and replied, "Ang, I know you want four kids, but Lucy and Gaetano are so small. There's no way I can risk getting pregnant again now. I'm already tired, and you know that you just have to touch me and I get pregnant." Angelo chuckled and said, "Ya, I know. Well then, why did we get a five bedroom house?" "I'm not saying that's it," I replied, " I'm saying let's hold off for a couple of years." Lucy and Gaetano were so close in age that it felt as though I had twins. I needed them to be a couple of years older before I even considered another child but for now it was not anywhere near my thoughts.

The day came for my appointment with Dr. Slater. I had no idea what to expect; the only thing I knew about IUD's was that I would not get pregnant. The doctor told me to take a deep breath and said, "Okay Antoinette you're about to feel a pinch." He was not kidding; I felt a sharp pain, and it felt as though he had stapled my skin together.

It was over in minutes, but I could feel blood trickling down. "You'll feel sore and you will bleed for a couple of days." He said. I did not mind the pain. The end results were worth it. For the first four months, I felt my left leg go numb and had trouble walking at times. I did not want to take the IUD out, because I did not want to have any accidents. After the four months though, the IUD settled in, and I did not have any more side effects. The IUD remained a part of me for over a year.

I remember going to a walk in clinic and saying, "I feel pregnant, but I know I'm not pregnant because I have an IUD." I waited in the patient's room patiently looking down the hallway, peering over at the nurse's counter where the stick that I had peed on lay. I kept thinking, "could it be possible, could I be pregnant?" but quickly put it out of my mind, reminding myself that I was being ridiculous. The nurse walked by and caught me looking over at the pregnancy test. She smiled and asked, "Is the suspense killing you?" I smiled and answered, "Yes." She picked up the white stick gently holding it between her finger and thumb and walked toward me.

She started to tease me, but her face went red when she looked down at the stick. "Do you have the IUD in you now?" she asked. I put my hands on my mouth shocked, "Yes, I do!" She held the stick up to my eyes. The stick was as purple as it was ever going to get, I was pregnant. We both started giggling. I was not sure what to think; all I knew was "here we go again."

I drove home, giggling all the way, but I am not sure if I was shocked or happy. I pulled into the driveway and just sat there watching Angelo on the porch. I parked the van, shutting the door behind me, and walked towards the porch, taking a deep breath I said, " I'm pregnant!" Angelo stood tall as can be and, with the biggest smile on his face, he ran down the steps to hug me.

I walked quickly into the house, not wanting to show Angelo my concerns and mixed emotions. "Maybe this is a good thing." I started thinking. "I can have the fourth child and I'll be done with child birth forever." But then, " The kids are so young, and I don't know if I can handle four kids under the age of five! On the other hand, they'll all grow up very close in age and they will like the same things." A tennis match went on in my mind, and every time the ball went one way I weighed all the pros and cons.

A final thought came to me, I became shaky and my stomach began to tense up. "My mesh, will my hernia come back? Can the mesh tear as my belly grows? How is this all going to work out?" I became very concerned and confused. I needed reassurance and grabbed the phone to call the doctor.

- 5 -
Our Home

I moved into Angelo's house once we were married. Angelo, along with his parents, had renovated an old, 1800 square foot home. They had installed wood flooring in all of the bedrooms and hallways. The main floor was covered with high gloss ceramic tiles. They hired people to build a bookshelf in the wall in the family room. The dining room was detailed to perfection with wall-to-wall cabinets and spot lights lighting up the china. I remember when my brother walked into the house for the first time. "Man, this house is a carpenter's dream." He said. Angelo had one of the bedrooms torn down to accommodate a large bathroom and a huge Jacuzzi, that was used often.

It was a lovely home and we lived in it comfortably for many years; but as the children came the house felt tight. The family room was filled with toys and I often had to tuck Joseph's toys in the corners. Joseph had his own room, that I had painted sky blue and trimmed its borders with airplanes. His queen sized bed was passed down to him from Angelo. Waiting for the arrival of his little brother Joseph felt like a big boy.

Gaetano received Joseph's nursery, painted purple with stars and moons trimming its borders. I sewed yellow curtains with purple stars and now all the bedrooms were occupied. I considered moving to a larger home, but Angelo would not hear of it. He would say, "We're comfortable here, besides, I love this house." "Angelo, there isn't any room for the boys to play." I would complain, I brought up the topic as often as I could, but Angelo dismissed the idea.

When I became pregnant with Lucy, I decided to try and convince Angelo one more time, "Ang, we need to create a room for the new baby, come upstairs with me." Angelo hesitantly walked up the stairs, while I waddled up behind him. I watched him go from room to room. I didn't have to say a word. I leaned on a wall with a smirk on my face as he turned around and said, "Okay, it's tight but we'll manage." I crossed my arms and replied, "How are we going to manage? Where do you want to put her, in the attic?" Angelo seemed confused. He bit his lower lip and finally said, "Okay, we'll look around for houses, BUT I'm not promising you anything." That was good enough for me. We drove around every weekend for months and fell in love with the suburbs. It was 45 minutes away from my family and two hours away from Angelo's, but the prices were reasonable and the houses were large.

Angelo still wasn't completely convinced he wanted to sell his first home. I had to push the situation a little further after all I was already eight months pregnant, but I knew the way to his heart. I fried up his favorite breaded veal cutlets and made pasta. When Angelo returned from a long day at work, we sat down to dinner. "Ang, I have a real estate agent coming to take a look at the house tomorrow." I began. I didn't dare look up and bit down hard on the veal in my mouth. He stopped eating and said, "You're really determined, aren't you?" I giggled and replied, "Well my girlfriend recommended him and I didn't think it would hurt to get an opinion on the price." Angelo shook his head and put a large piece of meat in his mouth. Savoring the flavor he swallowed and said, "Fine, I'll come home at noon to meet him. Make sure he's here at the same time." I clapped my hands, hopped off my chair, and leaning my arms around his shoulders, and kissed his cheek. "Step one completed." I thought.

The next morning I kept myself busy cleaning the house and keeping the children occupied. I prayed, "Oh God, please make this meeting go well." The agent introduced himself as Jeff, and Angelo said, "Come, I'll show you the house." As we walked around from room to room, I noticed that Jeff did not appear to be aggressive enough and I knew Angelo would take advantage of that. We returned to the kitchen, and Angelo spoke first, "Fine, if he can sell the house at my asking price, then hire him." I clenched my teeth and replied, "But honey, I still have another agent coming later this evening. We can let Jeff know our decision tomorrow. Okay?" Jeff stared at both of us, and Angelo said with a smirk, "No. Cancel the other guy and keep Jeff." Angelo said good-bye quickly and closed the door behind him before I could utter a word.

Jeff leaned over the kitchen counter and said, "You don't want me to sell your house, do you?" I answered quietly, "No." "Why not?" He asked. I looked up into his eyes and said, "Look Jeff, you're a great guy, but I don't need a nice guy to try and sell my house. I need a son-of-a-bitch, who will work like a bat out of hell, to sell this house as fast as he can. I don't want to give my husband a chance to re-think his decision. It has taken me a year to convince him to sell and I'm not going to have some nice guy screw it up for us." Jeff's face turned several shades of color, and I smiled as I watched it settle into tomato red. He became serious and said, "Give me four months and if I can't sell by then, I'll let you out of the contract. Deal?" I was very hesitant but said, "Okay, deal, but you have two months then you're gone." While Jeff did his best to bring in potential buyers, we put an offer in to the builders for our new 3100 square foot home.

Jeff came through; he sold our house in three weeks. Angelo changed all of the floor plans for our new home, and we fell in love with the design. This kept Angelo busy, and he did not fuss much over the sale of his home. We sold our house at the end of April, and on May first I gave birth to Lucy in a scheduled c-section. We had three months left in our house and I now had a new baby to tend to, a brand new c-section to nurse, and two little boys who needed my attention. Let's not forget, I also had a house to pack up for the move.

By the second week of May I had settled into a routine with all three children, and my hands were full. I got up in the morning and started my day with a large coffee. I gave the children breakfast and Lucy had her bottle. I put Lucy back in the basinet and settled the boys in front of their toys. I calculated the time between breakfast and lunch, so I would know exactly how much time I had for packing. I packed box after box marking each one. I served the children a sandwich and off I went back to packing. I became panicky when I realized Angelo would be home soon from work and I still hadn't started dinner.

I dragged myself into the kitchen and opened the cupboards searching for ideas for a quick dinner. I would think, "Off to the races I go, he'll be home soon." Angelo opened the back door and started laughing. I looked up and noticed his eyes were on the packed boxes. "Why are you laughing?" I asked. "Ant we have three months." He replied. "Are all the boxes full?" I smiled, "Yes." Angelo shook his head and laughing he managed to say, "you're incredible." I was pleased with myself and kept to my routine for months, day after day after day. By the time we moved in August, I felt a constant pain in my abdomen and I did not know what was causing it. Angelo kept telling me to see a doctor and finally I went.

- 6 -
The Mesh

The doctor pushed down on my belly, and I could feel a sting run from my belly to my back as he said, "I'm going to order an ultra sound just to be sure." I looked up and asked, "Sure of what?" The doctor was quite certain I had a surgical hernia. I waited for two weeks for the appointment; in the meantime I could not stand up straight. I felt a burning sensation, like the sting from a paper cut. I rubbed my abdomen constantly and tried to sooth the throbbing. The doctor called me after the ultra sound and confirmed I had a surgical hernia. My c-section had torn open from the heavy lifting I had done before and during the move. He referred me to a specialist and advised me to have it repaired. By October I could no longer stand the pain, and I knew I needed to have surgery. I had tried to avoid the operation because the children needed so much attention, and I wasn't sure how quickly I would heal.

The children kept me busy throughout the day. Joseph did arts and crafts every day, and Gaetano just wanted to touch everything in sight. I followed him all day, taking objects out of his hands, saying, "No." Lucy was becoming quite alert of her surroundings and required my attention. I catered to all their needs, but my hernia hurt more and more each day. I finally lost the battle and had the operation scheduled for late October.

The day came for my operation. Angelo had scheduled a couple of days off work. He headed to the van and I wasn't far behind. "I know everything will be alright, but just in case." I thought and quickly grabbed an old envelope off the kitchen counter and wrote in crayon, "Dear children never forget mommy loves you." I placed it on the counter and locked the front door. When we arrived at the hospital, I didn't feel scared or nervous, I just wanted to be done with it all. I put on the hospital gown the nurse had provided, and the surgeon came in to greet us, wearing blue hospital scrubs and a bandana covering his head. He was very tall and slender, and was confident and cheerful. "How long will the surgery take?" Angelo asked. The surgeon replied without hesitation, "No more than an hour. I'll just go in and sew her back up." Angelo and I didn't really have any concerns, so the doctor said he would see us later. I turned to Angelo, gave him a gentle kiss and said good-bye as I followed the nurse into the operating room.

Angelo bought a coffee in the cafeteria and waited for the hour to pass. He made his way to the waiting area where he tried to enjoy the weak coffee and pass the time. Minute after minute passed, then hour after hour. He paced the room and tried to make small talk with the people around him. When he noticed the hour was long gone, he began to worry and became anxious. He walked over to the nurses' station, "Excuse me, my wife's operation was supposed to take only an hour. Can you tell me if they're done?" The nurse picked up the phone and dialed. "I have the husband of Antoinette Romana wondering when his wife will be in recovery?" She said. She listened for a second then replied, "Okay, thank you." Her pretty green eyes were bright with a hint of eyeliner smudged at the corner. She looked directly at Angelo and said, "She's still in the OR." Angelo caught off guard by the news asked, "Is there a problem? Is my wife okay?" The nurse offered him a gentle and comforting smile, and said, "I'm sure everything's fine, I'll call you when she's in the recovery room."

Angelo thanked the nurse and walked away worried. "Did something go wrong?" he kept thinking as he walked back to his seat in the waiting room. Angelo purposely sat facing the clock and watched as every minute ticked away. His left knee shook quickly disturbing the people around him. "What the hell is going on? It's been four hours!" He thought and decided to demand some answers when he spotted the surgeon walking toward him. Angelo extended his hand and asked, "Is everything alright?" "I had to add a large mesh inside and sew the mesh layer-by-layer, starting from inside to the last layer that would close her up." The doctor replied and gave Angelo a reassuring smile. "Her recovery will take a few months.

Angelo came into the recovery room and took my hand with gentle strength. Tears covered my face and I could feel the pain. I felt as though all of my insides had been moved around. Angelo wiped away my tears and relayed the information the doctor had told him. I looked at him and asked, "What the hell is a mesh?" Angelo smiled and said, "It's like fish netting. They put a square piece into your stomach and sewed your inner layers of skin to it." I was completely surprised but at the moment I really did not care what they had done. My biggest concern was "When do I get the next morphine shot." I spent four days at the hospital and I recovered, in much pain, for the next eight months at home.

I remember Joseph at four years old taking a stepladder and putting it on the floor next to Lucy's crib. He would stand tall and pull her out, and then we would walk to the stairs while he struggled to carry Lucy in his arms. Joseph sat placing Lucy on his lap, and went down the stairs one step at a time, on his bum, while I followed backwards, guiding him, holding Gaetano's hand and helping him down the stairs. We did this for weeks. It was really very funny, and Joseph was so very proud of his good work, especially when I boasted about him to our family and friends.

- 7 -

Dangerous Position

"Would it all tear once the baby begins to grow?" I became anxious and called my gynecologist and told him that I was pregnant. I could feel his hesitation and I could hear paper shuffling in the background. "Don't you have the IUD in?" He asked, " Yes" I answered, my tone implying that this was his fault. After all, he was my doctor. He said not to worry and that he had performed four c-sections on the same woman before. I reminded him that I had a hernia repair and asked him if he had performed a c-section with a hernia in the equation. He hesitated then said, "Don't worry I'll have the surgeon assist me. You'll be okay." I still needed reassurance.

I called the surgeon that had repaired my hernia. He too was surprised to hear of my pregnancy and said that the mesh would have to be cut open and then repaired. "You and your husband should consider other options, because as the baby grows, the belly grows, and there's only so much stretching the mesh can offer. It could easily tear open and I am very concerned." He continued his advice, and stressed, "You're in a very dangerous position. Make your decision wisely."

I stood in the kitchen feeling completely annoyed and thought, "how dare he?" There was no other option. This baby is a gift from God. I'll just keep track of any burning sensations and try to get a lot of bed rest." I remembered that when the hernia had given me burning sensations, I would lie flat on my back and the aching would stop. "If I lie on my back like I did before it should be okay." I thought. I blew off the entire conversation. I was going to have the baby. Denial set in.

I called my mother. I knew it was going to be a bittersweet conversation. I put a smile on my face just before she answered the phone. I thought that if I sounded excited she would be excited too. It was more for her benefit than mine. When she answered the phone, I took a deep breath and said, "Ma, I have something to tell you." I waited a second and cheerfully said, "I'm pregnant." My mother did not say a word; I could hear her take a deep breath and exhale into the receiver. She did not think that my news was exciting; all she could say was "Mamma mia, how are you going to handle four bambini?" My smiling face did not work and I went into convincing mode, "But ma you had seven kids and you survived. Stop worrying." I could hear the intensity of her sighs and decided to end the conversation, "Ma, my other line is beeping. I've got to go, but I'll call you later." I did not give her a chance to say any more. I wanted to call someone that would be excited for us and not bring me down. After all, I needed some convincing myself.

Angelo came home and saw me on the phone. He started to laugh, "If you're going to let everyone know, then I'm going to make some calls too." He took the receiver out of my hand and made his first call. I could hear him trying to convince the person on the other end of the line. He kept repeating himself, "It will be fine." When he ended his call I took the receiver out of his hands started dialing the next lucky person. I received the same reaction as before, and tried to convince my sister we were happy about the news. I looked at Angelo and handed him the phone. We both laughed nervously. "I can't believe how worried everyone is." Angelo said. "What's everyone's problem?" I asked. He looked down at the phone and said, "I'm going to try one more call and then I'm done." Once again, he spent the next ten minutes reassuring his parents.

"What did they say?" I asked. "They expressed their concerns about finances, telling me I would have to work even harder now with four kids." He replied. I felt terrible for Angelo, because I knew he was very happy and wanted everyone to be as happy as he was. I put my arms around his waist and said, "You know what Ang? instead of five plates of pasta on the table we'll put six. Big deal." Angelo and I were ecstatic, and that was all that mattered.

We smiled for days, and I secretly spent a lot of time hoping it would be another girl, so it would even out our perfect family of two boys and one girl. I decided to name a baby girl Madeleina. I was very excited about the possibility that Lucy would have a sister. But if it were a boy, he would be named after Luca from the television series ER. I started to imagine my third son as a tall, dark, and handsome doctor.

Three months passed, and my first doctor's appointment arrived and all was well. I could already see my belly expand, and I walked around constantly rubbing it to comfort my baby. He seemed quiet in my belly, and I kept telling him, "Hey baby, you better be more aggressive than that, after all you have two big brothers and a strong-willed sister to compete with." I would start to giggle in hoping that he would move around more.

The doctor was in a good mood, "You know the drill, hop on the table." He was a thin tall man and always wore jeans and a shirt. His hair was turning slightly gray and he would always tease me and say, "My hair is going gray because I have four girls." He turned to face me, holding a bottle of jelly of which he dumped a bunch off onto my belly. It was very cold, and I could feel a chill go down my stomach. He placed a wand over the jelly and moved it around and around. I knew he was looking for the baby's heart beat. We could not hear a thing and Dr. Slater just said, "I guess it's just too soon."

Then Dr. Slater gave me an internal examination. I had dreaded this moment and hoped it would be over quickly. "The IUD attached itself to the sack, so we will just leave it in until the baby is born." He said. "Is this something to be concerned about?" I asked. He assured me it was fine.

"Have you been feeling okay?" He asked. "I am very tired. The kids really have me busy through the day, and with a big belly, well I'm just tired." I replied. I went on to say, " Of course I'm not as sick as I was with the other three. Dr. Slater this baby seems a lot quieter than the others. This pregnancy has just felt very different from the beginning."

He did not say anything and shrugged it off, while scheduling our next appointment. I just let it go figuring that I was overly concerned about nothing.

My sister Stella called and asked, "How did your doctor's appointment go?" I began with, "Okay". I could hear her breathing, but she did not say anything, and I knew she had bigger concerns. I finally said "Stella, what's on your mind? What are you worried about?" She wasted no time, and said "Is the doctor going to take the IUD out?" "No." I answered sarcastically. I could sense she was anxious, and could tell she chose her words carefully, "Anne, the doctor needs to take the IUD out, did you know it could cause Down syndrome?" I became very annoyed. I could feel my anger but assured her, "You're just being ridiculous "That wouldn't cause Downs. Besides the IUD can't be removed, because it would rip the sack." I ended our conversation quickly. After all, I always knew better than anyone else. Stella never mentioned it again.

The children knew I was having another baby, but Joseph was the only one who really understood. He was always very quiet and never shared his day at school with me.

Whenever I asked, "How was school today, Joseph?" He would answer the same, "Fine." I did not know he had told his class and his teacher about my pregnancy until one afternoon when I picked him up at school, a few mothers came over to me and said, "Congratulations, we didn't know you were pregnant." I looked at Gaetano standing next to me and Lucy in my arms. My eyes widened and I answered, "yup, I am." I had anticipated their sarcastic responses and it did not take long before one of the mothers said, "Oh my God, you're going to have very full hands." There it was, the comment I was waiting for. I had a rehearsed reply ready and said, "Yeah, my husband just can't keep his hands off me, and we're right on schedule, as planned."

I got up one morning happy and excited. I knew from the moment that I put my feet on the floor that, I was in the mood to spend money. I dressed the children and went to Wal-Mart. I stood in the baby isle for a long time trying to choose the prettiest baby book. I decided to buy a green book because I did not know the sex of the baby yet. It did not take long before the children complained that they wanted to leave. I picked a book with matching keepsake box and left the store ready to start filling it in. Once home, I fed the children lunch and sat them in front of their favorite television shows. I sat at the dining room table and started to think of all the wonderful information I could put in the new book. I began to write about how

I felt when I found out I was pregnant, how I told my husband, and what the names would be depending on the sex of the baby. I wrote down every little piece of information I could remember.

Christmas arrived and we had a wonderful holiday. Angelo gave me a Christmas card from the baby and the children, and we were so happy and excited. In the card he wrote, "I'm so proud to have such a wonderful wife, and the kids are lucky to have such a great mom." Tears formed in my eyes, and I moved the card around so I could see the words through my tears. He added, "The new baby is going to be very lucky to have such a great dad too." I laughed and read the card to the children. I gave them each a hug and a kiss and said, "You guys are so great!" My heart felt content knowing this was how my husband felt, and knowing my children felt safe.

Then came New Year's Eve and we went dancing with Angelo's parents and family. I remember telling my father-in-law that we wanted to name the baby Madeleina, for a girl, or Luca, for a boy. Angelo looked at me with a surprised look on his face and said, "I didn't know we decided on the names." I shrugged and tried to look cute, "You chose Joseph's name and Lucy's name. Now it's my turn." I smiled at him and focused my attention back to my in-laws. "All the Luca's I have ever known are mentally slow. I don't know what it is about this name but I don't like it." My father-in-law said, "Now Madeleina is a beautiful name. I like it a lot." He added. I did not worry about his comments. I loved the names I had chosen and let it slide. Later that evening I told my mother-in-law, "just think next New Year's I'll have four kids at this hall. I'll have to bring a playpen, so all of them can sleep if it gets too late". We all had smiles on our faces, and everyone danced till the wee hours of the night. The holidays were wonderful, but sadly it would be our last holiday together as the family we had known.

After the Christmas holidays, my in-laws left for a four month vacation in Venezuela, as they do every year. My mother was having terrible nightmares about me, which began to consume her days. My sister Stella kept calling and telling me, "Mommy is very scared of this pregnancy, she keeps dreaming that you die during childbirth." Stella kept hearing my mother say, "There is something bad about this pregnancy, and if she goes through with it, something will happen." I asked Stella, "Stella, what do you want me to do with this information?" "Nothing, I'm just saying mommy is very concerned." "Okay, I understand, but mom just has too much time on her hands." I was annoyed and did not know what she wanted to hear. At that point, even my mother's concerns seemed silly to me. I was on cloud nine, and nothing was going to scare me or concern me." Mom spends all her days worrying about me, and quite honestly, I think she is just bored. Focusing on me keeps her mind busy." I wanted no part of this conversation. "You know, I think you're right. Mom obsesses over you all the time." I was proud to be having four children. I reminded Stella of how wonderful it was to have so many siblings, and we began to reminisce.

- 8 -
An Italian Childhood

I had an amazing Italian childhood. My mother was a stay at home mom and my father worked hard at his barbershop. "Joe's Hollywood Barber Shop" I was so proud of the shop's name and I would often say to my friends, "Try topping that fabulous name!" I was the proud, spoiled baby of the family with one brother and five sisters. My father earned enough money to provide for us but we never had much, especially in the toy department. My sister Tracey and I would wait for rainy days so we could get our umbrellas out and go for a walk. Our mission was to go through the ally and steal toys left behind in back yards. We were always very proud of our new found treasures and we never dared let our mother or father find out.

When we were all together, I felt safe and happy. My twin sisters, Lina and Pina, were 16 years older than me, and often referred to me as their daughter. They were identical twins and I looked up to them until I grew up and realized that they were the shortest of my sisters. They were very cute with their dyed brassy hair and their big brown eyes. They were already married with children of their own by the time I was three. I was so excited when my sisters came over. I would sit at the kitchen table when they talked or just laughed. I would hang on to every word spoken and learn a lot about them. I do not ever remember hearing the twins ever utter foul language; the worst they would say was, "That fart." To this day I giggle when I think of the two women I referred to as "frick and frack."

My sister Maria is the third child, and she too was married and focused on her own family when I was a small child. Maria also dyed her hair a brassy blond and loved to keep her nails long. She was darker than the rest of us, and often commented, "I must be adopted." Maria is a strong willed and opinionated person with a good heart. I looked up to her as a child and tried to spend my days with her. In the summer, as soon as school ended in June, I would convince Maria to let me stay at her house, from July to the end of August. My mother would complain, "Antoinette, you need to come home. We miss you." But I always found an excuse to stay with Maria, and cried when I had to start school in September. Maria would cheer me up with a new outfit for my first day at school. I would wear my outfit with pride.

Stella was the fourth child. She was tall and like my other sisters, dyed her hair a brassy blond. Stella had her own room and filled her desk with makeup. I remember stories of how she used to model, but my father made her quit when she was asked to model bras in a television commercial. My father would not allow her to take part in showing off her assets on television, or anywhere else, for that matter. From then on her modeling career was over. As for me, well, I would sneak into Stella's room when she was at work and would very carefully put her make-up on and pretend to be her. I often thought of how beautiful she was and wanted to mimic her. She remained in my parents' home until she married, when I was eleven.

Finally my mother had a boy to carry on the family name. My father was very proud of his son and showed him off to everyone. Guy was four years older than me, and I always respected him, my only brother. Guy was tall and slim, with dark black hair and big brown eyes. He always pushed me to be the best I could be and often pushed me to my limits. I remember making myself a sandwich after school, and Guy licked it so I could not eat it. Once he took me to the nearby high school and told me to run the track. I was a chubby child and Guy wanted better for me. I often laugh over these stories, because he really was quite obsessive about my weight and he loved me enough to care.

Then there was Tracey. She was two and a half years older than me. Like Maria, she too had a dark complexion. She had long black hair, and, unlike me, she was very thin and always a bit taller than me. Tracey and I were the last two girls at home and we were close. We played together all the time and spent a lot of our time being mischievous. Inevitably, we would fight a lot, and, those were the funniest times.

Once we were arguing, and I chased her around the house, yelling, "I'm going to kill you." Tracey, who was always considered smarter than me, locked herself in the washroom. This time, however, she wasn't going to outwit me. I took the insect repellent spray that my mother hid in the closet and ran to the washroom. If you don't come out, I'm going to kill you like a cockroach." I said and waited, but Tracey would not come out, so I did what I had to do. I sprayed the bottom of the door, and the spray went through the crack. Tracey started choking and climbed up on top of the sink to open the window. I ran outside under the stairs, to spray the window. My mother came running and could not believe her eyes. She started yelling, "Are you crazy? You'll kill her. Give me the bottle." As she ripped the bottle out of my hand, she smacked me on the side of my head and yelled, "get in the house."

We heard a loud crash, as we entered the kitchen and mom ran toward the washroom. Tracey opened the door, and I could hear her cry. Tracey was soaking wet, her hands in the air, and her tears poured down. My mother looked over her shoulder and yelled, "Call your father and tell him to shut the water valve!" I peeked into the washroom and saw the white ceramic sink on the floor in two pieces. Water poured from the pipe, and I knew I was in big trouble. Tracey stood yelling, "The sink broke off of the wall when I tried to climb down." Then headed toward me, screaming, "You bitch, you tried to kill me." I ran as fast as I could, but my nervous laughter slowed me down. My father was furious when he saw the mess, and spent two days to repair it.

My father never had much to offer us, but we never lacked in love. He never drank or smoked, and he never went out with friends, but he had many acquaintances from his barbershop. When we wanted to go horseback riding my father would take us to a friend's farm where we rode donkeys. We did not know the difference but we had so much fun. In the summer we would all go to Boyd Conservation and spend Sundays at the beach. In the winter, my father would make an ice rink in the back yard, and we would get second hand skates. My father taught us how to skate and fend for ourselves. He would often show Guy how to fix things around the house, and my mother taught us how to cook and clean. She would often say, "You need to learn all these things, because one day you will have to take care of your own family." My mother often pulled Tracey and me away from the television and ordered us to watch her cook. She would teach us about the different spices and explained how important it was to have a lot of flavor in our food. That was just the way it was ... Perfect.

Stella and I had reminisced for hours that day when she remembered that she had to pick her son up at school. "Did I ever tell you what dad said to me about my marks?" I asked. "No, but you have to tell me the story quickly." I began to recall that we did not experience a lot of pressure to do our schoolwork. The only person who was pressured to have good marks was Guy. We all knew that Guy would have to find a good job to provide for his family one day.

I began, "One year we brought home our report cards and daddy had to sign them. Well, he looked at Tracey's report card and said "bravo Pappa" signed it, and off she went. Then he looked at Guy's report card. He was pleased with the marks and he again said, "bravo Pappa" and signed it. It was now time for my report card. I really wasn't very good in school, no matter how hard I tried, but I passed my report card to daddy. He looked at my marks and said "ats ok Pappa when you growd up, you get married and have bambini." that was that and I went to play." Stella started laughing, and said, "Is that what daddy said?" "yup." I answered I love this memory because it really was all I ever wanted, and now I had it, I had it all. Stella and I laughed every time we reminded each other of all the good times we had growing up. Finally, we said at the same time, "Okay I have to go." I had to get dinner started, and look for the kids.

- 9 -

An Amniocentesis

February 9th, 2004, Dr. Slater had ordered the usual blood work and an amniocentesis because of my age. I asked him if the amnio was necessary, and he replied, "I don't offer my patients a choice." I challenged him, "Why not? if someone doesn't believe in abortion, what would be the purpose of this test?"

He seemed annoyed and said, "If that's the case, you should have the test done, so you can educate yourself if there is a problem before the baby comes." He continued, "In all my 30 years, I have never had a patient who has chosen to keep the baby when it was diagnosed with Down syndrome." I was quite surprised with his answer, but did not dare to challenge him. I had had an amnio done twice before, and I honestly thought it was not a big deal. I just did not want to go through the motions once again, after all, I had three healthy children, why would this be any different.... or so I thought. I never thought for a minute that my world would soon change forever.

The hospital called a few days later. I anticipated the call so I was not surprised to hear the woman on the other end of the line. "Hi Antoinette, I am calling from the genetics department. Dr. Slater has ordered an amnio for you. I have a date for you on February 18, 2004." I wrote the date down on the calendar on the fridge, and thanked her.

Angelo came home that evening and washed up for dinner. I told him the date of the amnio and said, "Book that day off work, so you can take me to the city. God knows, if I attempt to go to the city alone, I'll end up in Timbuktu." Angelo nodded and said, "Make sure you arrange for a sitter." Later that evening, I finished up the dishes and called my mother, "My amnio test is coming up and I need a baby sitter." I knew that whenever I needed something I could call my mother with my concerns, and she would make a round of calls for me. Not an hour had passed, Angelo and I settled down for an evening of watching television, while the children played around us, and Maria called "Mom said you needed a baby sitter for a few hours." I smiled, "Yeah, but I won't be gone for too long." "Bring the kids to my place for that day." She offered. I knew my mother would come through, I chuckled as we hung up.

The days passed and I was getting closer to the scheduled date for the amnio. Angelo and I were not concerned about it; we were happy and carefree. I wrote the date of the amnio on the baby's first year book and got ahead of myself and wrote, "Three weeks have passed and everything is just fine." Stella came over for a coffee during the week. "Are you concerned about the amnio at all?" she asked. "No, not at all. By the way, Angelo and I were going to ask you and Lui to baptize the baby." I replied. Stella took a sip of her coffee and said, "That's great. We would be honored. I can't wait to go home and tell Lui." "Don't announce it to anyone until the amnio is over. After all we wouldn't want to jinx ourselves." I told her.

Every once in a while, I thought, "could there really be anything wrong?" but I never thought it could happen. After all, growing up I always thought that if you did not look at a sick person, it will not happen to you. I remember when I was pregnant with Joseph, if I saw a Downs person or an autistic person, I would look away quickly so I wouldn't get their cooties. My thoughts were ridiculous, and yet I justified my actions by telling myself, "Everyone does the same thing, they just don't admit it." Having a Downs child was my biggest fear, and I would have followed any superstition or drank any potion to save myself from what I was about to experience.

When I was growing up, I always ran away from my fears. As a child, I would fake being sick just to avoid a test or a project at school, and my mother never questioned me. In grade six, my gym teacher made me captain, for an afternoon, of a mini soccer game. I was already at school and could not play sick. I was so afraid of being the leader, I started shaking, and the fear of God was in me for the entire hour. I really did feel sick and I thought I was going to vomit. I tried to tell the teacher, but he just said, "Get out there and start playing, then if you still feel sick I'll call your mom." Every minute we played seemed to last for hours, and I asked God to help me through it. The game went well, and I was very happy when it was over. Someone called out the score, but I did not hear them nor did I really care.

The day came for my amnio. We rose early and were in a great mood. The children ate breakfast, I was dressed, and Angelo was still asleep. As I was waiting for the coffee to percolate I recalled what my mother-in-law once said. Angelo and I were engaged and were looking for a hall for the reception. We had booked an appointment to see a hall on a Friday night and asked Angelo's parents to come with us. Angelo and his father both smoked, so they sat in the front with the windows partly opened. Angelo's mother and I comfortably sat in the back. Music was playing, and Angelo was having a conversation with his father. We could not hear what they were saying, so I sang along with the song on the radio.

Angelo's mother leaned over and said, "You know Angelo has never needed for anything. I have always taken care of anything he needed." I looked at her and said, "Yes, I know." "Not for anything, I have always washed his clothes and I have his dinner ready every night." She stressed. I smiled and said, "Yes, I know." "Angelo doesn't know how to fend for himself. He wouldn't even be able to sew a button on his shirt." She continued. I smiled at her lovingly and said, "I am prepared to do all these things for him." "Don't forget to bring an espresso to him in bed every morning, it helps him to wake up." his mother added. She waited for my reaction and said, "I have always woken him up with an espresso. I would like for him to have what he is accustomed to." I smiled and said, "Yes, I know." I just never knew how tedious this task would become after many years. The coffee was now ready and I served it to Angelo in bed.

We got in the van, and of course, the usual conversation came up; there was no gas. Angelo was at his wits end. "Do you ever put gas in the van? Ever?" and my reply, as always, was the same. "You don't do indoors, and I don't do outdoors." We both started laughing, and Angelo held my hand tightly, shaking his head. On our way to the highway we passed two gas stations, and I told Angelo, "Get gas." But he of course, answered, "We'll get it off the highway." Going south bound on the high way I kept telling him, "Ang, the gas tank is below the red line now." I became anxious, and my teeth were beginning to grind. He only smirked, and said, "Don't worry."

I knew he kept driving to put the fear in me, so I would start getting gas when it was needed. I do not think he expected it to run out so quickly. No sooner had he uttered those words, he started slowing down and pulled over to the shoulder. The nasty part of it was that we could see a gas station right ahead.

I became very nervous and could feel my stomach tense up. I knew that now we would be late. Angelo would have to walk along the highway to the gas station for gas. As soon as the driver's door closed I started praying Angelo would be all right. Joseph and Gaetano started to ask, "What's going on?" Well, Joseph did, Gaetano just wanted to know if daddy was going after the aliens. We started singing songs to stay busy, and I kept track of the time. "We're going to be late. Oh God is this some kind of sign. Do you want me to miss this appointment? Oh God, please don't make us be late."

I looked up at the rear view mirror and saw the statue of the saint surrounded by a white wheel hanging there. I put my hand around it and said "Hey dad, watch over us and please have Angelo get back soon." My father always had this saint in every car he ever drove. He said the saint protected us on the road and would guide us. I came to believe in the power of this little statue as well.

A red pick up truck pulled up next to us and I was scared for a split second until I saw Angelo jump out from the passenger door. He was carrying a red gasoline jug. He shook the driver's hand and the man drove away. In my head I said, "Thank God, thanks dad." The kids cheered for their father and continued with their songs. I looked at Angelo and said, "That was faster than I had expected." "The man was a really nice guy. He offered me a ride back to make it faster." Angelo said. We were back on the highway but I knew we were going to be late.

Angelo drove as fast as he could. We cringed at every red light and cheered at every green light. On yellow lights we took our chances and ran through them whenever it was safe to do so. We made it to Maria's house. "Where were you guys? Why are you so late?" She asked. I rushed the children in the door "Long story. I'll tell you what

Angelo did later." I smirked as I passed Angelo. He was helping me get the baby bags from the van and laughed, "Ya me, you can't put gas in the car." "Sorry. That's your job." I said and we both started to laugh. Angelo tugged at my shoulders and pushed me out the door. I gave Maria quick instructions, after all Lucy and Gaetano were still in diapers. "Naps, don't forget to give the kids a nap by 2:00 pm. I yelled before we drove off. Joseph will touch everything, he needs to be carefully watched." Maria told me to stop worrying, "Go, go, don't be late and take your time."

My mind jumped from one topic to another. I kept thinking, "We are going to be so late." then, "That's a big needle I'm about to get shoved into my belly." I felt nervous and anxious. Angelo interrupted my thoughts, "Call the hospital and tell them we're on the way." I called Dr. Slater's office and the secretary said, "Hold and I'll call," While I waited, Angelo and I talked about the sex of the baby. The secretary came back on the line and said the department was not answering, we should just go and pray for the best.

The ride felt as though it took forever even though there were no traffic lights on the highway. Finally, we saw the hospital sign up ahead and we knew it would not be long. Angelo dropped me off at the emergency doors and went to park the van while I waited in the lobby. When he came through the doors, he took my hand and kissed me with his warm lips and we walked to the information counter. Angelo kept teasing me, "You're about to get a huge needle!" I shook my head from side to side, stuck my tongue out slightly and said, "bla bla bla." Angelo was very pleased with himself and smiled.

As we sat waiting in the department, a slim young girl came toward us. She was a pretty blond with hair down to her shoulders; she couldn't have been more than 25 years old. She spoke very softly, and extended her hand to greet us. "My name is Jane, the pre-screening counselor. It's very nice to meet the both of you." Follow me." We went to her office where she pulled out some forms for us to sign. She began to ask, "How many children do I have?" Angelo replied, "three." "What are their ages?" "five, two and one." I replied. Jane started to smirk and said, "I'll bet your hands are full!" "Yup." Angelo and I replied at the same time. In between her questions, Angelo made jokes about how potent he was or how many more times he was going to get me pregnant. Jane played along and said, "Angelo you're really funny." I just kept thinking, "Gee, I wonder how funny it would be if I was shoving the needle in him." But I never uttered a word; I just giggled at his jokes, they really were funny.

Jane said there was just one more thing to do and that was to call downstairs and let them know we were here. She made the call and all we heard was "What? No way. Well they're here already. Well, can he be paged in the parking lot? Please try and get back to me." Oh my God, another sign from God I thought. Jane explained that the doctor performing the procedure had left, and that they were going to try to get him back. Jane kept her composure the entire time, but I could tell she was worried. She held the door open and said, "You can both wait in the lounge, and

I'll find out what's going on." Angelo and I were heading for the lounge when he looked back and said, "Please do something. She's too many weeks ahead and we will be too late for any rescheduling." Jane's soft blue eyes widened and her pale face turned a brighter pink. She said quietly, "I know. I'll do everything I can."

Angelo and I sat in big brown tub chairs in the lobby, and I could see Angelo's mind racing. I always knew when he was deep in thought, because he would bite his lower lip. I kept staring at my watch, knowing that every second mattered. "Ang, it'll be okay." I said, but that was not what I was really thinking, which was, "Oh shit, this is not good." The more I stared at my watch, the slower the time went. It felt as though every minute took an extra 20 minutes to pass. I decided to turn to a higher power and I started praying to Suora Anna Maria Rosa. I asked her, "Please guide this day, and if this amnio is meant to be, please help the situation." Those were my words, but my thoughts, quite honestly, were "Please have the doctor come back."

Suora Anna Maria Rosa was a special nun in Italy. She was my aunt's roommate. My aunt Zia Ida was also a nun from the time she was a young woman. Zia Ida would always tell us of the little miracles Suora Anna Maria Rosa performed. Whenever we felt down or scared, my mother encouraged us to pray to Suora Anna Maria Rosa and ask her to help us give our fear up to her and to God. My mother gave me a ring many years ago that belonged to Suora Anna Maria Rosa. She told me to wear this ring whenever I needed guidance, and I believed in my mother's words.

I sat in the big brown chair, twirling the ring around and around and recalled the day I put that ring through a test. Years earlier I was in a terrible relationship and I knew I did not want to stay with this man any longer. My mother kept telling me to leave him. She was afraid we would get married, but frankly, I was not so sure. I remember putting the ring on and asking Suora Anna Maria Rosa, "Please make things better for us, please have him change." That very night he called, and I could tell he was not coming to visit because he was slurring his words. He was completely drunk.

I kept the ring on my finger and held my hand over my head. I stared up at the ceiling and said, "You know what, Suora Anna Maria Rosa, you can all shove it. None of you are listening to me. I'm done." I went to my bed and fell asleep crying. The next morning, I woke up and my hand was shaking and trembling uncontrollably. I knew at that moment Suora Anna Maria Rosa wanted the ring off my finger. I tore the ring off and said, "OKAY, it's off." My hand stopped shaking, and I knew she was angry with me. I told my mother what had happened, and she said, "She's angry because you didn't listen. She gave you an answer, but you didn't like her answer." I knew at that moment she really was listening to me and I needed to understand her.

After that lesson, I believed in Suora Anna Maria Rosa's miracles. I do believe in how powerful prayer is and right now I need that power.

Jane came back and said, "The doctor came back. Come on, we must run. He is waiting." We jumped out of our seats and headed toward the elevator. I could see the relief in Angelo's face. He looked at me lovingly and we did not have to say a word, we both knew what the other was thinking. Another nurse met us and quickly told me to change into a robe while Angelo waited outside. When I came out, she said the doctor was waiting and Angelo and I walked in together. The room was painted gray and the light was very dim. There was a desk by the door and a bed in the center of the room with a computer screen next to it. I knew this room well. I had been in here twice before. But although the room was the same, the doctor was not. He was an elderly man with a small gray mustache and gray hair; he had kind piercing blue eyes and a warm smile. "Thank you for coming back. I was really worried for a minute." I said, and Angelo pretty much repeated my words, he truly was grateful.

The nurse rolled my gown up to my chest and started applying a cold gel all over my belly. Fear started kicking in again. I just did not want a big needle, but having been through this before, I knew it would be over quickly. She started moving the wand around and around my belly as she faced the screen, looked for fluid in the embryonic sack. Angelo began asking a million questions. He was dying to know the sex of the baby, but she could not tell because the baby was moving around too much.

I looked over and saw the shadow of my baby sucking its thumb. Delighted and excited, I kept saying, "Oh my God, he's sucking his thumb." The doctor poked my belly very gently, pointed the needle down and said, "Okay Antoinette, when I count to three take a deep breath in and let the needle gently glide. Whatever you do, don't move; we don't want to poke the baby we just want the fluid sitting in the sack." The procedure took only about 60 seconds, and I was very happy when it was over. The nurse wiped the jelly off and told me to keep my feet up for the rest of the day. So now the worst part is over, and I will never see this room ever again….. Or so I thought!

I got dressed and went into another room where a volunteer handed me a glass of juice and guided me toward a reclining chair. Angelo came over to pull the lever for me. I gratefully sipped the juice, while the volunteer monitored me. In the mean time, other women came in and did the same. Angelo spoke with the other husbands about their children, and of course, Angelo is so proud of his children that he can go on forever. I love listening to him. He is such a proud man and speaks so highly of us.

When the volunteer came back and said, "Okay, Antoinette you're free to go." Angelo said good-bye to his new friends and off we went. Slowly we headed back to our van holding hands. I made sure to take my time, so I would not develop cramps. Arriving at Maria's house, I could hear the children yelling, "Mommy's home!" They did not give me time to come in the door, and jumped up and down, grabbing on to my legs. I was so happy to see them and was ready to go home. "Come in for an espresso."

Maria said, I told her about the procedure, "I'm so glad it's over. I always cringe when that needle starts to go in." "Did the doctor say everything's okay?" Maria asked. "We won't know for a couple of weeks. I'm sure everything's fine."

The next day, we returned to our regular routine with no interruptions, and the days that followed were the same. Gaetano and Lucy had their bottles on schedule and their diapers changed. Everyday Joseph asked, "Mommy can we have arts and crafts?" We filled the hours with decorative projects and all of my attention was placed on the children. The children loved finger painting, and it was always a challenge to keep the paint on the paper or at least on their hands. The paint spread all over the floor and the smiles on their faces were priceless. I would put all three of them in a bath and watch them play. The kids had crayon soap and they colored each other in different colors. I sat next to them and thought, "Well, the hospital hasn't called in three days, so I guess everything's okay." I smiled at the thought of my four children as I dried them.

I let the children play with their toys and sat down to pay bills as quickly as possible, knowing that I needed time to get dinner on the table. I looked at the calendar on the fridge and said, "Oh ya, today's almost over. Another day not to worry about the amnio." I looked down at my belly and rubbed it, thinking, "This baby never really moves around much." Dinner was cooked slowly on the stove and I was exhausted. I decided to lie down on the sofa. I lay on my back and rubbed my tummy and said, "Guys, let's sing a song to the baby." The children sang the theme from

Barney and I joined in, hoping the baby would hear my voice and move around.

That evening I told Angelo, "This baby seems so different from the others, he's very quiet and doesn't move. We even tried singing to him today." Angelo rubbed my belly and said, "Good, finally we'll have a quiet child that takes after me." I punched his arm and turned around to sleep. A large part of me knew that something did not feel right, but I just told myself, "Everything is fine, I'm just being paranoid." Looking back, I thank God for this. I think it would have been even harder on me, had the baby reached out to me in that way.

- 10 -
Angelo And Me

After I received Jane's call, I sat at the kitchen table and thought, "I knew there was a reason I couldn't sleep last night. I just knew it." I sat, wiping my tears away with my hands, and waited for Jane to schedule my baby's death. From where I sat, I could see the end of my brown wooden table and the antique gold colored walls. I looked over at the hutch that proudly displayed my china. But now the china meant nothing to me. I would smash it all up, if it would change something. The sliding doors were shut to keep the cold wind out and I stared out into the backyard, watching the trees sway back and forth. I could not help thinking, "I need air." I was having trouble breathing and every tear that fell seemed heavy. I could feel my heart breaking, but it did not cleanse me. It felt as though sharp pieces of glass chipped away from my heart.

I had often heard the term, "broken heart." but I never realized that with every tear a piece of my heart came through. No one I know could ever say that they knew how I felt and I pray to God that they never do. Yes, this loss was my choice, but it was more devastating to me, because Angelo and I had chosen it.

I walked over to the sliding door and stood outside in the cold. The wind had pushed its way into my bones and I shivered, but did not dare to move. I pleaded with God and cried, "If you could just have me miscarry right now, so the choice would be yours not mine." I held my hands together over my eyes and tried to continue, but the prayers would not come. I was overcome with rage, my face became hot and the heat burned through my skin. My stomach tensed up and I looked up at the pale blue sky. White clouds moved quickly, and I felt my sense of heaven run away from me. I stared at the clouds and screamed, "Why God? why me? Why are you allowing this to happen to me?" The rage poured into my soul. I slammed my hands on my chest. I wanted an answer from God and I wanted his explanation then and there. I stared at the moving clouds and said, "You cowards run, go ahead, run." I looked at the trees and watched them blow hard. I lowered my head and yelled to God, "Fine, you left me with my very own cross to bear and I'll bear it, but you're going to help me carry it."

The phone rang. Jane said, "I have booked the procedure for March third." She stopped for a moment, and I knew she could hear me whimpering. She continued, "I've booked you at the abortion clinic, because if you choose to have the procedure done at the hospital, you will have to be induced and go through labor." I was taken aback by her comment and said, "What do you mean?" "Well, it's against the law to have an abortion at the hospital. What we do is, induce the labor early." "Oh my God, no, no I just can't." I interrupted her. "I think the abortion clinic will be the best way for you to go." She said.

I was silent for a moment, then, said with composure. "Okay that's fine." My head was spinning, and I could not believe I had just said "fine". What the hell was so fine about it? I used this word as though I was ordering a damn coffee, and they ran out of sweetener and offered me sugar instead. "Come to my office at 8:00 am for counseling, and then you and Angelo can drive to the clinic". Jane said. I had so many questions but could not think of one at that moment. Jane seemed ready to end our conversation, but I was not. I did not want to hang up. She was in control of the situation, and I needed her to make all the decisions; I just could not do this alone but I said, "Good –bye." and put the receiver down with great hesitation.

"Oh my God, Angelo doesn't know yet." I buried my face in my hands and thought about this sweet beautiful man, this gentle soul who tries to help everyone and asks for nothing in return, except for his coffee in bed every morning. I smiled when I thought of him. Angelo shows such great love for me and our children and our extended families. He always shows great respect to our parents. I will never forget how kind and gentle he was to my father right up to the day he died.

My father no longer had the strength to do the smallest tasks for himself. We all chipped in to help feed him and help him get dressed. Angelo and I had been dating for a few months by then and we spent a lot of time with my father. We were watching television and my father was anxious. I could tell something was on his mind. "What's wrong pa, what do you need?" He looked at me with such frustration and said, "My beard, I need to shave my beard." Angelo did not hesitate for a second. He jumped up from the sofa and said, "I can shave you." My father looked at him with a big smile and nodded, accepting Angelo's kind offer. My mother was pleased, "Let's get him to the washroom, and you can shave him there." I offered to get my father's electric razor. I felt so proud of my boyfriend and thought, "If he can make a man he barely knows this happy, I could only imagine how he would love his wife and children." Angelo took his time with my father that day and made sure he shaved every inch of his face. After that day, my father called on Angelo to shave him whenever it was needed. I never once heard Angelo hesitate to help my father and I never hesitated when I fell madly in love with Angelo.

Angelo always believes the cup is half full and he is always intent on teaching people to see each other's side of any story. He never speaks poorly of anyone and he always tells me to do the same. Our love for each other is very intense. We have enormous respect for each other, and I cannot imagine my life without him. "We love our children more than our own breath, but when they grow up and leave our roof, it's just me and you, babe." I always tell him. Angelo never hesitates to hug and grab me. I love to push him back and say, "Angelo, I'm busy right now." He pins me in a corner and says, "But I love you. Wanna go upstairs for a quicky?" Looking so pleased with himself, and I began to laugh and push him just enough to duck under his arm and escape, "You're such a scurvy dog." I say. Angelo always makes me smile, and I feel so safe and happy with him.

We always consider each other in every decision we make, and the friendship we have is like no other I have known. Now, I will break my best friends heart; I am the bearer of horrible news. I tried to picture his reaction and this brought me back to a conversation we had years ago when we were dating.

Our relationship had gotten pretty serious, and we knew we were meant to be together. It was a Saturday night, and Angelo said, "Let's go to the drive in." He drove a black Daytona, which he was very proud of, and I always felt very cool when I sat in his fancy sports car. Angelo paid for the tickets and drove around forever, trying to find the best spot for a full view of the big screen. I wore a tiny blue summer dress with buttons down the front and the cutest blue sandals with a small heel. I felt sexy and cute.

"I've got a great idea, come with me." Angelo said. I always cringed when Angelo got an idea, because I knew it meant I would have to follow. He opened his door and reached into the back seat for a blanket. "Angelo, I would rather sit in the car and watch the movie from here." I said. "No, this will be really great. Just come" "But Ang, I'm wearing a dress and heels!" I argued. He walked over to my side of the car and opened the door giving me no choice. He held his hand out and I got out of the car. With great hesitation, I followed him to a chain that separated the grass from the pavement. Angelo had strong long legs and climbed over the chain without a struggle. He grabbed me by the waist, and I tucked my feet under my bum, while he pulled me over the chain.

"Oh God, I'm gonna break my neck." I thought and wondered how many people watched us, calling us idiots. Angelo looked so happy as he put the blanket on the grass and lay on it. "Isn't this great, we can watch the movie under the stars. Come on lie down with me." I bit my lower lip and lay down next to him, trying to like it.

Angelo suddenly became frantic and started flapping his hands around his head. "It's a swarm of mosquitoes." He yelled. Before I could jump up, I was being attacked too. Angelo grabbed the blanket with one hand knocking me off. I had no choice but to roll onto the grass. I bolted toward the car. Angelo had a longer stride and ran faster than I ever could, and I tried to keep up. His strong long legs jumped over the chain, and I tried to follow but my heel got caught in the chain and I could feel the tug. "Oh God, here I go" I cried out, and down I went. Angelo turned back and with both hands around my waist pulled me up. I had such a disgusted look on my face when I heard Angelo laugh uncontrollably and I stared him down. He tried to avoid eye contact and picked up my sandal giggling.

The heel had broken off my sandal, and I wanted to start laughing, but did not dare, I was too busy pretending to be furious. I was relieved when we got back to the car and closed the doors. We both caught our breath, and I waited for Angelo's next brilliant idea. "It'll be a while before the show starts. Let's put the back rests down and get comfortable." He said.

We began to talk about our families and our future. "Angelo, all I ever wanted was to get married and have children." "Would you stay home or do you want to work?" he asked. "Oh, definitely stay home. I want to raise my own children. Do you think a woman should stay home with the kids?" "Yeah, no wife of mine is going to work, that's my job to provide the bacon." I loved his answer, it was exactly what I wanted to hear. "How many kids do you think we should have?" he asked, "I always wanted four." A beautiful smile came over his face.

Angelo placed his hand on my cheek and leaned forward to kiss me. His kiss was warm, and I could feel his strength as his lips tugged at mine. I felt so tingly inside and I did not mind if our embrace lasted a long time. "What if we found out our baby had Down syndrome or something like that? Would you abort it?" Angelo asked. I did not expect his question, it came out of nowhere, but I knew it was a valid question that needed to be addressed. " Well, I really don't believe in abortion, but a special needs child would be a difficult situation." I answered. "What if we knew the quality of life wasn't bright for the baby, would you then?" he asked. "I guess so, but that's not going to happen to us okay?" I sat up and pulled the backrest back to an upright position.

When I looked into the parking lot, my eyes grew wide. "Angelo look." "What the hell?" We both burst out laughing and looked at the clock. It was well past 2:00 am, and there was not a soul to be seen or a car to be spotted. The lot was empty, and the movies were over. The evening had been wonderful, but little did we know that our free and easy conversation would one day come to bite us in the ass.

- 11 -

Decisions

I kept trying to brush away the tears so I could dial Angelo's number at work. When his beautiful voice answered, I could sense a smile come over his face, and his voice was cheery "Hey baby, what's up?" I took a deep breath so the words would come out clearly but as I exhaled the tears pushed their way through and took over. "Ang, Jane called from genetics." I stopped and a muffled sound came out, "the baby has Downs syndrome." I could not catch my breath, my heart pounded and I kept thinking, "How the hell do I spare the pain for him. How can I take his pain and deal with this alone." I wanted to spare him every bit of this information, but I also knew that I needed him to get through this moment. Angelo was silent for a couple of seconds. I could hear his heavy breathing through the receiver. I waited as he tried to register the words. "Oh baby, I'm on my way." He said gently. I heard the receiver being put down and the line went dead.

I was still holding the receiver when Joseph walked into the room. He tugged on my sleeve and said "mommy why are you crying?" I pulled him onto my lap, looked into his beautiful big brown chocolate eyes and said, "because I hurt my finger." He placed my hand in his tiny little fingers and asked me which one. I smiled at his beautiful little round face and wiggled my baby finger. Joseph brought down his strawberry red lips and gently kissed my finger. "Thank you baby, now I feel much better." He jumped off my lap and walked away contently, not knowing how broken I felt inside. I stared at him walk."Thank you God, I needed that." I thought. "Maybe we can do this. If we have a lot of help, I'm sure I can find a support group that can guide us." I thought out loud. A thousand ideas brushed through my head. "Could it be possible?" I tried to think of the positive, but then my thoughts moved on to the scary side, "How will we manage. What if all the pressure destroys our family?"

I was so confused and I did not have any idea which way to go. I needed Angelo to come home and tell me what to do. I knew he would guide me to the right decision. I tried to sweep the floor and keep myself busy until he came home. I needed to call someone. I needed to scream and cry to anyone. Our families needed to know what was happening, and, anyway I was never good at keeping my personal business to myself. I needed everyone's full attention right now. Most importantly, I needed to hear that I was making the right decision. I called Stella. I barely gave her a chance to say hello before my words came pouring out. "I got a call from Jane." I said. "Calm down. Who's Jane?" she asked. "She's from the hospital. She said the baby has Down syndrome." Stella's voice became soft and I could hear her sadness come through. She tried to encourage me. "Focus on your kids and pray." "Are the tests 100 % correct?" she asked. "ya." "I'm coming over. I'll see you in a bit."

Next, I needed to talk to my mother. I needed to know what she would do in this situation. We were on the phone for quite a while, and my mother remained very calm. She just kept telling me, "Leave it all in the hands of God and pray to Suora Anna Maria Rosa for guidance." I kept arguing, "Oh ya, Suora Anna Maria Rosa. Do you think she's going to make it all better? How about God? No, I know I'll pray to dad. Do you think he can make it all better with a wand?" She tried to understand my pain, but her love for God is great and she believed I could get through this with his help, "Just ask God to take your pain." I do not know whether her chanting helped or got on my nerves. It was not my mother's words though; it was my anger with God, my anger with everyone I pray to. After all, does God not make these kinds of decisions? As far as I was concerned, God handed me this problem, and I was not about to let him off the hook easily. I was also angry with myself, angry with my body and angry at my soul.

Angelo walked in the door and I ran to him. As soon as I saw the sadness in his face, I said, "My God, what have I done." I told him the news over the phone. I had not considered that he had been driving home, trying to register the news." "Thank God, you made it home safely." I stared at his face. I needed to make sure he did not hate me. I needed confirmation of his love for me. He did not say a word, but put his arms around me and held me tight.

My head fell on his chest, and I felt my whole body fall into him. His sweet smell went right through me, and I knew that one day we would look back at this, knowing we got through it together. Our bond was stronger than ever, and I could feel his heart pound.

His first words were "Are they sure, could there have been a mistake?" Tears began forming in my eyes, "There is no mistake. Jane from genetics said the blood work that Dr. Slater ordered was positive, and the amnio confirmed it; they checked the results twice." His eyes were sad and intense, and his face was flush. I could sense his disappointment and sadness, but there was nothing I could do for him, there was nothing I could do for myself.

Stella arrived at my door not 10 minutes after Angelo. She kissed Angelo hello and asked, "How are you doing, Angelo?" "I'm okay." He replied. They followed me into the kitchen. "Anne you're making the right decision, you've got three small kids you need to worry about." Stella said. I sat down on a bar chair facing her as she began cleaning the counters. I honestly did not hear a word she said, my mind wandered off. I did not know what to expect and I was scared and confused. I kept thinking, "Does a fetus feel everything?" At one point I looked up and saw

Angelo and Stella staring at me. "She's in shock," Stella said and Angelo nodded in agreement. The phone kept ringing but Stella and Angelo answered all the calls. I do not remember taking care of the kids or making dinner or even when Stella left that night. I felt as though my mind had left my body and wandered away. Angelo went back to work the next day, but his boss told him to go back home and take the following week off. I do not remember him at home and, quite honestly I cannot remember anything from the following 72 hours. I had no choice but to take care of chores and I had three children to tend to. While I took care of their needs, I was constantly on the phone going over and over the information and putting myself through hell. At the end of the day I would ask myself, "Did I eat today? What did I cook?" My thoughts would turn to the children, "Did the children have a good day? Did they eat enough? What did they eat?" I did not have answers to any of my questions. I wanted to be in control, but I just did not have the strength. For the next few days, I woke up and cried, I went to bed crying, and I cried, pretty much, all day, every day.

Dr. Slater called, "I received the report of the amnio and I want to know if you booked the appointment for the procedure," "I did." I answered and began to cry. "Antoinette you don't need this in your life. Go ahead and take care of it, and next month, I'll tie your tubes." His voice was neutral, as though he had said these words a million times before. I choked back my tears and asked, "what's its sex?" "a boy" he answered sternly.

Many calls from family and friends started pouring in. For the most part everyone tried to be supportive and listened to me cry. Each had their own way of consoling me, but there were no magic words to stop me from crying. Some had different beliefs and were not afraid to express them.

The phone rang. "It's the overseas operator for Mrs. Antoinette Romana." "That's me." I replied, "I have a call from Maria." I knew that Maria was down south on vacation, but I was surprised she called. "Anne, I just got off the phone with mom. She said there's a problem with the baby. What's happening?" I started crying and told her, "Mar, you're not going to believe it. The baby has Down's." I reached over to grab a tissue, my nose was dripping. "Anne, I figured that much by mom's voice. Listen, I am backing you up 100%. You have no idea how hard this life is. I'm more afraid that you may consider keeping it. Anne, please be strong and let it go." "I'm not going to reconsider, but I don't understand what happened." I replied. Maria's voice remained calm and stern, "Anne, stay strong I'm going to call you every day." I was about to hang up when I heard my niece Carm's voice on the phone. "Hi Anne, are you okay?" "Not really." I cried. "You're doing the right thing. I'm heading to the church right now with my mom, and we're going to say the rosary for you. Be strong and we'll call tomorrow." Carm said.

The phone rang constantly, and I never contemplated letting the answering machine pick up. Every call was my chance to repeat my sad news over and over again. As soon as I ended a call, the phone would ring before I even put the receiver down. As I began to speak, I had already forgotten whom I had just spoken to or what we talked about. I repeated Jane's words to every new voice and tried to figure out if they were on my side or not. I felt a sense of relief when I heard the words, "I would have done the same thing." When I heard hesitation in the caller's voice I defended myself and stated my case. My stomach would tense up and I felt like vomiting. I never tired of telling everyone every bit of my private and personal details. I spent hour after hour on the phone crying, but the tears did not make me feel better; they just tired me out enough to reach the feeling I longed for. I wanted to feel numb. I never realized that crying on my family's shoulders would later on work against me.

One morning a relative called. "Hi Ant, how are you feeling?" "I'm just so tired." I answered. "What are the kids doing?" She asked. I had no idea where the children were and I walked into the playroom before I answered, "They're just playing with their toys." "Ant, I've been thinking about your situation." "Ya?" "I would respect any decision you make because I'm not in your shoes." "Aha." "Would you consider giving it up for adoption instead of having an abortion?" I gave it a moment's thought and answered; " I don't think I could ever forgive myself for abandoning him. I'm not giving him up, because I don't want to raise him. I just worry about his quality of life." She interrupted me, "But maybe someone else knows how to raise a Down's child." At this point I became annoyed and said, "I don't think this is an option." My eyes swelled up with tears. My words came out chokingly and I could not speak any longer. "I didn't mean to upset you, I just want you to consider every option."

I sat down at the dining room table, leaned over and buried my head in my crossed arms. "How the hell do I live with myself, knowing I've abandoned my child to a stranger. No. I'd rather give him back to God." I thought, I dismissed the option completely, but not until I ran to Angelo and told him. Angelo just shook his head and said, "Don't think about it."

The next caller started with, "I have a friend who has a Down's child." "Ya?" "Do you think you may want to speak to her?" she asked. "What for?" I answered "So you could get a better feel for the situation." "Thank you, but the decision has been made, and I am already confused as it is." I said. I did not want to speak to her friend. "The thought is appreciated. Please tell your friend thank you anyway." "I hope your not offended by my call." She replied. "No. I'm not offended." "Do you think I should call her back and tell her I changed my mind?" I asked Angelo. he took a sip of his coffee, "I'm sure everything is fine right now. Tell her to talk to us when her kid is grown up." I could hear the frustration in Angelo's voice and walked away saying, "You're right."

The day quickly turned into afternoon, and I tried to start dinner. I pulled a pot out of the pantry and thought, "My God, I haven't checked on the kids for hours." "Thank God Angelo's home." I said out loud. He had kept an eye on the children for most of the day. I went to the playroom and held up some fish crackers in a plastic bowl. I shook the bowl and said, "Who wants a snack?" The children had been playing happily with their toys, Lucy and Gaetano dropped everything and yelled, "Me." I placed the bowl beside them. and watched them push a couple of crackers at a time into their mouths. I could see the sadness in Joseph's face. "What's wrong baby?" I asked. He did not look up and just replied, "Nothing." I was about to ask again, but the phone rang again.

"Hi Ant, how are you feeling." Again I said, "I'm okay, just tired." She tried to make small talk, and I could hear in her voice that she had something to say. My stomach tensed up and I finally said, "So what do you think of this entire situation?" At that very moment, I wanted to kick myself. I knew no good could come out of that question, but I never know when to shut up. I could hear in her voice that she had prepared an answer. "Well, I only believe in abortion if it is rape." I laughed and said, "Oh, so when it's rape it's not a baby?" She said, "Ya, it's a baby but..." I tuned her out completely and thought, "My God, you're an idiot. I wonder how long you practiced that one?" I considered telling Angelo, but then decided this call did not merit repeating or getting upset over.

The calls kept coming well into the evening and began first thing the next morning. My first call was from my cousin," I don't quite agree with your decision. If you choose to keep the baby I can help out." She said. "Thank you for offering a solution. You're the only person who has offered, but we've made our decision." I replied, but I wanted to consider the possibility of outside help.

I decided to ask Jane what she thought. "Hi Antoinette, what can I do for you?" Jane asked cheerfully. I could hear the clicking sound of the keyboard. "Do you think that with the help of family, just maybe I could handle it?" I asked. Jane sighed and the typing stopped. I knew I had her full attention. Her voice became sympathetic, "Antoinette, if you chose to keep the baby, you can only depend on yourself. Angelo would have to work to pay the bills, and as good as everyone's intentions are," She hesitated and continued, "it's like a death. Everyone is around for the first month, then they go back to their own lives, and the help is gone." For a moment I had had a shred of hope, but now I felt shattered once again. I had wanted Jane to tell me it was a great idea, but that did not happen. Now I needed to re-think everything all over again and come up with a new plan. At the very least I had to convince myself once again that we made the right decision to let our baby go.

I wiped away my tears and answered the phone once again. It was a relative of Angelo's. "Did Angelo tell you I called yesterday?" She asked immediately "Ya, he said he spoke to you." I answered. "Well, I don't know if he told you about our conversation or not, but I told Angelo, if you don't want to raise a baby with Down's, I will raise him for you." I was shocked, my hands trembled and my face became as red as a pepper. I wanted to call her every vicious word I could think of, but I held my tongue and answered, "I wouldn't give you any of my children. Down's or not." "I'm just offering you an option." She replied. "You couldn't offer him a normal life any more than I can." I said. She tried to cut in, but I continued, "I can't believe you would call and say this." My body began to shake, and I knew I was about to cry. I told myself, "Don't give her the satisfaction of crying." When we hung up I was hysterical.

I called Jane once again and repeated every word. Her voice became angry "In all my years as a counselor, I have never heard such a ridiculous comment." I sobbed into the phone as she continued, "Antoinette, people don't think when they talk, you're going to hear it all. You will need to learn to brush off all the ignorance." With every breath I sucked in, I was able to get out a word, "Do you think I don't want to raise him because he's sick?" "It doesn't matter what I think, or what anyone else thinks. You need to do what's best for you and your family. I know you are making the right decision. Think of your three kids." She answered. I thanked her once again for her time and she said, "Listen, you can call me as many times as you need."

Angelo could see the anger in my eyes and asked, "What's wrong?" With my hands on my waist I said, "Why didn't you tell me about last night's conversation?" "I didn't want to upset you. I knew her comment was dumb and I just decided to ignore it." Angelo said. "Thanks for the warning." I said as I walked away. I tried to tidy the kitchen, but could not shake my anger. All of the phone calls began to get on my nerves. I needed to calm down. "Watch the kids, I'm going to lie down for an hour." I told Angelo, I did not wait for his response and went upstairs as the phone rang once again.

I lay in bed with my eyes closed, but paid close attention to Angelo talking on the phone. I knew Angelo tried to whisper so I could sleep, but I could hear him explain the situation to someone. I knew by his words that he was speaking to his parents in Venezuela. Angelo came running up the stairs and said, "I know your tired but my parents want to talk to you." I sat up and took the receiver from Angelo "Hello?" "Antonietta, stay strong. We support you and we agree with your decision." My mother-in-law said, I started to cry and said, "Ma, can you believe it?" "I know, just go with your decision and don't turn back." She said, I began to sob as she spoke, "I had a good friend years ago that had a Down's child in Italy, and both he and his wife grew old really fast in the years from all the worries." She repeated, "Be strong." I could hear the phone exchanging hands and then I heard my father-in-law, "Antonietta, just don't look when it comes. Don't look, because that memory will be edged in your mind forever." I said through my tears, "Thanks dad." He continued, "God is with you." I could not talk anymore and I passed the phone to Angelo.

Angelo's voice cracked as he spoke to his father. I could not hear what they were discussing, nor did I try. Angelo talked to his parents for a long time as he wandered from room to room. When he wandered back to our bedroom, I heard him say, "I am really hurt from the lack of support given to me." He wandered off to another room, and I decided to leave that conversation between Angelo and his parents. I could feel Angelo's tears in each word he spoke. I knew that if I went to him, he would hold it all in, trying to remain strong for me. This was the first time I heard his sadness and I knew he was really hurting.

I could not sleep thinking of Angelo. I tossed and turned and found myself facing him. I stared at this beautiful selfless man. He looked so peaceful lying on his side. I kept thinking, "I'm being so selfish. I know you're in pain too." I needed him to feel my warmth and leaned over to kiss his lips gently. I did not want to wake him, but a part of me wanted him to feel my kiss. He felt the warm embrace and opened his eyes. "What's going on?" He said and he rubbed his eyes, trying to see through the darkness. I leaned into him and said, "Ang, I love you." He stretched his arms over to me and, with a gentle tug, put his arms around me. Angelo pulled me closer and said, "Oh baby, this sucks." I laughed and said, "What, that I love you?" Angelo smirked and replied, "No this entire situation." I did not want to talk about it. I just wanted to know he still loved me and to reassure him that I still loved him. I buried my head in his chest and whispered, "Make love to me." Angelo gently took my hands and held them tight as he lay on top of me.

We took our time and appreciated every moment of our lovemaking. I knew our lives had changed forever and, now I discovered, so did our passion. We followed every curve of each other's body with our fingertips, and Angelo's kisses were sweeter and kinder. I did not want to rush and embraced his caresses. He kept whispering, "I love you." and I absorbed every word like a sponge. I did not worry about tomorrow, my only thoughts were the here and now and I did not want it to end.

We lay next to each other and watched the daylight slowly creep into our bedroom. "I don't want to deal with

another day. Can't we just go back to last night?" I said.
Angelo smiled and gently caressed my face with his hand.
He leaned forward and kissed my lips.

He looked into my eyes and said, " Ant, stop listening to
everyone. They all have their opinions, but in the end this
is our life, our decision, and our family to take care of." I
tucked my body in closer to him and said, "I know." I felt a
little better that morning. Our close bond from the night
helped me find more strength within me, strength that I
needed to find. My body had felt beaten and broken. Now,
I felt at peace. Angelo proved to me that our tragedy had
made our love for each other stronger than ever. I felt his
strength that night and knew we were facing this together.
It was not just me.

I made the children bacon and eggs. Lucy and Gaetano
bickered at the table, and Joseph remained very quiet.
Angelo and I enjoyed a cup of espresso while we wiped
the egg yoke from their clothes. "Do you want me to put
on your favorite movie? I asked Joseph, He answered in a
very low tone, "No." Everyone scattered around the house,
the children found toys they enjoyed in their playroom
while Angelo found the television remote. I, on the other
hand, needed to talk on the phone.

I thought I would call Stella and have a light conversation.
But it was inevitable, I began to talk about our problem
again. "Stella, you won't believe some of the comments
I'm getting!" I became uptight all over again. My stomach
tensed up and butterflies were flying around my tummy
once again. I could hear the anger in my words "People

are so stupid. I spent the entire day crying over their comments." Stella interrupted me and said, "Anne, stop worrying about everyone else. God is the only one you Needed to confirm your actions to." "I know, but it's so hard." I went on to say, "How the hell do I forgive myself?" "Find a way. The only thing you're guilty of, is trying to save a child from a hard cruel life." Stella replied. "I was talking to mom last night and she made a really good point." she continued, "Mom said, tell Ant, to cry for the next 30 days, but at least you won't be crying for the next 30 years." "Oh, I don't know about that." I said. "By the way, mom's bad dreams about you have stopped". Stella said. "That's good. I know she was convinced the dreams were happening for a reason." my voice began to crack, and I could feel tears coming on. "Anne, are you crying?" "I'm trying not to, but it just happens." I replied. "Well if it makes you feel better then cry.

I lay on the sofa for hours staring at the television. I had to convince myself to change the children's diapers and make morning snacks for everyone. My mind was in overdrive, and I spent hours trying to find a way to justify our decisions. "My God, tomorrow I am about to go through with the abortion and I can't find a valid reason to go through with it." I kept thinking, "Maybe I should go talk to the priest. After all, he's the closest I'm going to get to God." I began to cry, "On the other hand, abortion is against our catholic religion. What if the priest disagrees with Angelo and me? No, I must go. I need to know what a priest would say." I walked over to Angelo and said, "Ang, there's an evening mass at 5:30 tonight." Angelo looked up at me without saying a word. "Why don't we

all go to mass?" I suggested. "Whatever you want baby."
He replied. I felt pleased and answered, "Good. I'll get the
kids dressed."

I rehearsed what I would say to the priest, practicing over
and over, changing my words and trying sympathetic
phrases. I could not find a way to guarantee the priest
would be on my side and I could not risk him being against
us. "Okay I'll just ask him to pray with us." I decided. The
children were not used to going to church, and I knew
they would get bored. "Let's sit in the back." Angelo said.
I agreed and gave the children some dry cheerios to keep
them busy. "I really need to bring the kids to church more
often." I thought. As the mass continued, I saw Angelo
deep in thought. I leaned into him and said, "Ang, you
don't have to come with me to speak to the priest." "Are
you sure?" I smiled and said, "Ya, it's okay. Don't worry
about it." I was enjoying the prayers, but at the same time
I felt anxious and still had no idea what I was going to say
to the priest.

After mass, I was directed to the priest's office and waited
in a chair for a couple of minutes, thinking, "I wonder if
I'm going to talk to the same priest from mass." No sooner
did my thought end, the priest walked into the room. He
was a short stalky man, with black greasy hair and a round
face, and he wore his long black gown. He pulled up a
seat and asked, "What can I do for you?" I was about to
spill the entire story onto his lap, when there it was, a big
silver cross with Jesus nailed to it. The cross was attached
to a beige rope around the priest's neck. I could see God
looking at me with a disgusted look on his face, saying,

"See what happened to me," I felt as though I had been slapped in the face.

I looked up, the priest sat in his chair staring at me, waiting for me to tell him why I was there, but I could not do it. I sat back in my chair and said, "My baby is sick, and the doctors need to abort the fetus." "Okay, technically his health can't be saved." I was thinking. As the priest began talking, I just tuned him out and went into my own world. I kept thinking, "Oh God, I just lied to a priest." When he finished talking, I said, "Thank you, father." I ran out of his office as fast as I could.

"Thank God, that's over." "I have no idea what that accomplished." I told Angelo. As we drove home, I decided that I only needed to get God's forgiveness for our choices. From now on, I would pray directly to God.

- 12 -
Parting from Luca

"Today is Monday. Oh God, Today is Monday." I sat up in bed wiping away the tears. I rubbed my belly and cried, "I'm sorry Luca, please forgive me." I wanted the baby to feel my embrace. "You're going to be happier with God, I promise." Angelo walked into the bedroom and said, "I heard you crying, are you okay?" I put my feet on the floor and replied, "No. I just want today to go away." Angelo came over and brushed my hair with his hands. I wiped my tears and hurried downstairs. I knew we had to leave the house soon and I was frantic.

My mother had made arrangements with Stella to come and watch the children. The doorbell rang, and I looked at the clock on the stove. It was 7:00 am, and I thought, "Good, they're right on time." I heard Stella take her shoes off and my mother shuffle her walker around. I walked into the hallway to greet them and mother' looked very sad. "We should get going." Angelo said. I grabbed my purse and said, "There's food in the fridge. Cook whatever you want for the kids." Stella put her hands on my shoulders and gently pushed me toward the door, "You don't have to give me instructions. I know what to do."

I was grateful, because my mind was not on the children and I felt confused. Angelo and I were somber. We kissed the children good-bye. "Mommy, are you going bye bye?" Lucy asked, "Mommy will come home soon."

I kissed Gaetano and looked at Joseph. I walked toward him, but he quickly leaned up against the wall. I bent down and said, "I'll be home soon. I love you so much." I put my arms around him for a hug, but he did not reciprocate. I stood up quickly holding my breath. A burst of tears plunged through me and I did not want Joseph to see. My mother and Stella gave us hugs and said, "Be strong. God will provide."

The drive to the hospital seemed long and gave both of us time to think. I felt my heart pound in my chest as I cried. "I can't believe this is happening." My arms and shoulders felt tense and very heavy. My temples pounded and I knew that releasing my tears would tire me out for a while. Angelo held my hand, but did not say a word. He spent the entire time biting his lower lip. I tried to find something comforting to say to him, but I just could not find the words. I took the time to tell my baby, "I'm sorry." "Wouldn't it be neat if we got to the hospital, and Jane tells us she was looking at someone else's file all this time and that there was nothing wrong with Luca." I said to Angelo. He glanced at me and said, "Ant, don't do this to yourself." I turned away from him and stared out the window. I tried to return to reality, but I needed peace, even for a short while, in the shape of denial.

We got to the hospital, parked the car, and went straight to Jane's office holding hands. "Come in." She looked at us with her piercing blue eyes and acknowledged me with a small smile, "How are you doing?" I looked at her but I could not answer. Angelo and I sat down and waited for Jane's next move. She pulled out a brown folder and said, "I'm going to show you your report. This will show you the numbers the lab used to determines Down's." "What if we go through all this and the lab is wrong?" Angelo asked. Jane gave us a soft smile and said, "The reports are not wrong. Angelo, I know this is hard to understand, but you have to face reality." There was a knock on the door and a woman walked in. She was tall lady and a slightly heavy set. She seemed very professional and introduced herself, "I am Dr. Lewis." "Doctor Lewis has worked with Down syndrome patients for over 30 years." Jane said.

I was anxious and hoped, "Maybe this doctor could shed some light on the entire situation." My big brown eyes focused on her face, and I waited for her to notice my desperation. I kept hoping that if she could see my pleading eyes, she would give me hope and change the outcome. "I'm sorry for what you're going through. As bad as this all seams right now, you are making the right decision." Her voice was low and very matter of fact. I became angry; I had heard those words a thousand times before. I kept thinking, "Tell me something I don't know." My anger turned into tears, tears for the words I did not hear. Dr. Lewis leaned forward and placed her hands on top of mine. "Antoinette, Down's children are very cute kids. They are the most loving people and their love is unconditional. They do the best they can in school and they are happy, but the reality is, when they grow up they're not so cute any more... they are lost souls." As she spoke I did not want to look at her, even though she was on my side.

I felt ashamed in the presence of a doctor but a larger part of me wanted her pity. I kept thinking, "If an educated doctor is telling me to abort, maybe my decision, is correct." I stared at her soft white hands, her plain gold wedding band and the diamond ring next to it. The diamond sparkled and I tried to concentrate on how many rainbow colors I could discern in the light shimmering on it.

I heard Angelo's voice crack and I looked over at him. I knew he had his own questions and I was curious as to what questions had not yet been asked. Angelo's eyes went from Jane to the doctor, and I just knew he was looking for hope. "Could this report be wrong?" he asked. The doctor immediately shook her head from side to side and gave him a small smile. His one little glimpse of hope was once again shattered, when the doctor said, "No." Jane opened the beige folder in front of her, pulled out a sheet of paper and passed it over to Angelo. I glimpsed over his arm and saw a map. It had directions to the abortion clinic. I turned away quickly thinking that if I did not look at the words, I would not have to go to that disgusting place.

"I'll call you in a couple of days to see how you are doing." Jane said. We all stood up. Angelo looked at the doctor, his hazel green eyes now shiny from the tears he wanted so badly to let flow, and kept a steady glare.

Angelo and I did not say a word the entire drive, and there was a somber feeling between us. I was numb at the thought of our destination and could not believe where we were headed. My mind was screaming, and the car felt like a big cage that I could not escape from. "How the hell do I enter the doors of death? Oh my God, I'm such a hypocrite; I have made the wrong decision. This place isn't for me." I crossed my arms around my waist and thought, "This place is for sluts and whores. It's for people who don't love God or his creation. I can't be here. I'm a middle class housewife. I'm a good person. I don't belong in there." I pictured the clinic painted in black and everyone there walking around like zombies. I felt scared and alone but what was more frightening was that I would become one of them.

Angelo parked the car at the side of the building. I was glad because I did not want anyone to see me enter the building, not even a stranger. I knew Angelo thought the same way and that he was carrying shame with him as well. He confirmed it when he grabbed my hand and led me to the back doors. Once again I knew I was not in this alone and I felt safe. We walked up two flights of stairs. At the top of the stairs there was a heavy metal door with a red a sign, RING DOOR BELL. Angelo rang the bell and we waited. I looked around and the seriousness of the place was apparent from the security they practiced.

A voice spoke through the intercom, "Good afternoon, may I help you?" I was surprised at the sweet sound of her voice. I leaned into the intercom, "My name is Antoinette Romana and I have an appointment today." "Okay, just a moment."

Angelo silently pulled me into his arms. My tears fell onto his jacket, and every tear was riddled with guilt. "I'm so sorry Ang, I'm sorry my body screwed up." I meant what I said; I knew it was all my fault. I kept thinking that if he had married someone younger, this may not have happened to him. He pulled me closer and said, "It's not your fault. God is punishing me." Confused I moved away from him. I thought quickly, if he springs something bad on me like an affair or something, I am going to ask the clinic to put me out of my misery and kill me too. "God's getting me back for all the girls I fooled around with when I was single, and bad choices I made as a teenager when it came to the girls." He said. I felt a huge sense of relief and exhaled. We looked at each other, and I started to laugh. "What's so funny?" Angelo asked. I felt happy for a split second and said, "Okay I'll accept that answer. It's your fault."

A buzzer went off, and the door opened. The room was painted a pale beige, there were pamphlets on the wall and a desk by the door. I caught a glimpse of a large room filled with women and a few men. I did not notice anyone's face except for that of the woman behind the desk. She did not seem to have red horns sticking out from the top of her head nor did she wear a black gown. She was just a normal person, and somehow I was disappointed she gave us no excuse to get the hell out of there. She looked up at me and with her soft blue eyes and said, "Have a seat."

I was so embarrassed to be amongst the crowd of all these "lovely" people. I kept my head down in shame and tried not to catch anyone's eye. "Look at all these low lifes." I thought. I did not allow myself to imagine their stories. I was trial and jury in a second's glance without knowing anything about them. There was so much casual chattering going on around the room, it annoyed me.

Nearby sat a young woman who could not have been more than 16 years old. She wore skin tight jeans, and her runners were tied loosely on her feet. Her frame was petite as was her little black t-shirt. She sat back in her seat with her legs crossed and read a magazine with an older woman, I assumed was her mother "I wonder how good a mom you must be." I thought. They were discussing fashion trends and pointing at models in the magazine. I could not sit still and commented to Angelo, "You would think this place would be riddled with remorse, ha?" Angelo took my hand and said, "Let's not judge."

I could not help but nit pick everyone in the room, after all, I was nothing like them. I was a woman of circumstance. I continued to look around the room to find my next victim, and there she was, a young woman sharing a story about a party she went to the previous night with a few of her friends. I wanted to walk over to her and say, "Hello, anyone home? Do you get why you're here?" I bit my tongue. No one seemed very sad about what they were about to do.

On the other side of the room sat a tiny Chinese woman. She was so petite and had long straight black hair. She seemed young, but wrinkles from stress lined her face and she looked to be about my age. Her Asian eyes were glossy with tears. An Asian man sat next to her, and I assumed he was her husband, because he had the same desperate look that Angelo had. I caught her staring at me, and we gave each other a small smile. I wondered what she was thinking, but then again we both knew why we were there, and our sad smiles painted the entire picture. I knew at that moment that my judgment of others only served to make me feel better. "I wish I could go over to her and find out her story. Maybe we can console each other." I thought. "I can't stand this any longer." I told Angelo. I tried not to think of the Asian woman and focused on the others. It was easier to judge them than the woman who mirrored my story.

A woman holding files in her hand walked into the room and said in a loud voice, "Antoinette?" Names were called out and we stood up. I could see the disappointment of those who were not called, but I did not care. We followed the nurse into a tiny room. A doctor introduced herself to me and said, "I just need to review your file." She asked me about my hernia and spent a lot of the time taking notes. She then put her pen down and looked up at me. We locked eyes with very serious looks on our faces. She began to explain the procedure, "We place something that looks like a balloon with a liquid in it; then we place it into the uterus. From there you go home and you may miscarry during the night; if not you come back, and we'll give you a clean up here."

90

Her words were cold. My heart pounded and I imagined that the thumps were from the baby knocking, screaming, "No, please no." It all sounded confusing, but even worse, it all sounded final. "I can't do this." I said to Angelo. He just looked at me, but before he could say anything to comfort me, another woman came to me and said, "You need to change into this gown for an ultrasound." I could not look at Angelo. I stood up and walked away with the nurse. I could hear the woman at the desk tell Angelo to wait in the waiting room. I was about to go through this alone.

I lay on a table for the ultrasound and I could not control my feelings. I needed Angelo to be by my side, he was the only one that really understood our grief. I started crying uncontrollably, and the nurse rubbed my leg. "Is the baby sick?" She asked. I nodded and said, "Yes." "Everything is going to be all right." She assured me. I felt that she knew I was not like the others in the waiting room and I felt her compassion for my choices.

As I watched the nurse pour jelly on my stomach, I held my breath at the thought of seeing my baby on the screen. For this short time, I knew that my son was safe and warm. "Maybe he hasn't felt my crying or my fear. Maybe he is sucking his thumb and loving the sound of my heart beat." I turned to look at the computer screen with a sick feeling in the pit of my stomach, and yet with excitement. I wanted to catch a glimpse of him, but the nurse turned the screen away from me. I did not have the courage or the strength to fight her decision. "Maybe I have given up the right to see him, maybe I deserve this punishment." I turned my head back to the center of the room. My mind kept telling me to say something. "Can you." But before I was able to finish my sentence the nurse grabbed a cloth and said, "There, we're done." I felt robbed of a moment I could have had with Luca and was mad at myself for my weakness. The nurse knew this moment would have only been filled with remorse. "Maybe it's for the best." I comforted myself. Part of me was glad I wasn't given the option.

I wiped my tears away and was escorted into a small room. There were a handful of women sitting there, all wearing the same gown as me. I found a seat in the corner and wondered what was next. There was a chill in the air and I folded my arms as goose bumps began to form on my legs and arms. My teeth chattered as I sat there with my eyes facing down. All I could think was, "Maybe I should have done this at the hospital. I don't want it to be this way. Oh God, please help me." No sooner did I think these words, a nurse came to me and said " Antoinette, get dressed the counselor wants to talk to you." Her voice took me out of my trance, and I quickly stood up. I found the cubicle with my clothes and got dressed. "What the hell is going on?" I felt as though I was back in school and was sent to the principal's office to be reprimanded. The anticipation was overwhelming. Angelo was already sitting there when I walked in. We looked into each other's eyes confused.

The counselor laced her fingers together and placed her hands on the table. She looked at me with bright blue eyes and said, "Okay, we have reviewed your medical history, and quite frankly the clinic is not a hospital. We are very concerned about your hernia repair." Angelo sat up and asked, "So what are you saying?" "We do not want to perform the procedure." I felt panicky. Was this another sign from God? "If something were to happen to you," She continued, "we do not have the medical equipment to help you. I'm sorry Antoinette, I suggest that both of you call the hospital and speak to your counselor."

"I never want to see you or this place ever again. Good riddance." I thought. Angelo and I got our coats and walked out. I could feel the tension in my shoulders start to relax, and the butterflies in my stomach fly away as each step I took distanced me further away from the clinic. "Let's just go home. Maybe this wasn't meant to be, Ang, let's go home." I could taste my desire for Angelo to agree, but he looked into my eyes and said, "We can't turn back now." I grabbed the sleeve of his jacket, forcing him to pay attention to me. "Please Ang, we need to go home, please." My voice began to crack even though I knew what needed to be done. Angelo's eyes were glossy with tears he fought so hard to hold them back. He quickly dialed the hospital. "Can you please connect me to Jane in genetics." I felt tired and defeated and was grateful for Angelo's strength. "Ant, Jane said to come straight to the hospital. She said she wants to talk to us." I could see in Angelo's eyes he was desperate and I knew he too needed direction. I wanted to get angry and put my foot down and just go home, but Jane and Angelo had taken over the situation, and frankly, I was grateful.

Being with Angelo always made me feel safe, especially when I could not handle a situation, I knew he would take over. His strength reminded me of our honeymoon when we drove through Europe for 33 days. Angelo did the driving and I was the navigator. I could not read a map to save my life and Angelo knew it. "Just keep the map open and follow the highway. You need to get us to Paris."

We started in Germany and I followed the lines on the map with my orange highlighter. I was not about to give Angelo any sense of satisfaction. I thought I was doing well and was quite proud of myself. When we were tired we stopped at a little gift shop off the highway. I began to wander around the store and picked up a pair of wooden shoes. "Why would a little gift shop in Paris sell little wooden shoes from Holland?" I asked, and we started to laugh. When we got to the counter Angelo asked, "Can I please have a map of Paris" The young girl behind the counter replied, "We only have maps of Holland." Angelo looked at me then back at her, "Where exactly are we?" "You are in Holland" "Honey, we're in Holland." I laughed so hard that I could not catch my breath. I crossed my legs, desperate not to pee, "This is your fault. I was not kidding when I said I couldn't read a map." Angelo laughed and said, "I'm taking over." Thank God. That's exactly what I wanted to hear and I left it all up to him.

Years later I was, once again, relieved to leave it all to Angelo. At the hospital we were escorted to a private waiting room where we waited for Jane. The walls were painted peach, and had two chairs that were arranged by a desk with a computer. Angelo turned the computer on and logged on to the Internet; he began a search on Down syndrome. There was an intense look on his face;

he needed to see our situation in black and white. A part of me wanted to know as well. I got up to peer over his shoulders and saw pictures of children with Down's. They all had big smiles on their faces and seemed so happy. Angelo quickly moved on to the medical information. There was much to read on the heart problems and bad vision they have. Angelo muttered, "I can't believe how little we know about down's." His thirst for information propelled him further. I did not want to read any longer. I returned to my seat and said, "Ang, just turn it off."

Jane walked in and said, "Hey guys, I heard from the clinic." "What do we do?" Angelo asked. "Come with me, we'll talk." Angelo and I followed Jane to her office. We found a number of people sitting around a table there. I sighed deeply in disgust. As soon as I saw the doctor from the morning, I realized that this was to be an intervention. I thought, "Angelo must have told Jane that I wanted to change my mind."

I sat next to Angelo and a woman I did not know sat to my left. She said, "Antoinette, I too am a counselor at this hospital. We just want to make sure you have all the facts you need to make a decision that's right for you and your family." They did not hesitate for a moment; the doctor's voice became quite stern. She raised her voice and I had no choice but to focus on her words. "Let's get down to the bare facts. Antoinette do you have at least $150,000.00 put away in your bank account?" Confused I answered, "No." The doctor continued, "Well that's about how much money you're going to need if this child needs to be put in a home." She paused for a moment allowing me to digest the information. "You're already 38, lets say you die at 70, your son will be in his 30's, who do you think will take care of him? Your daughter wont, after all, she will have her own husband and children to take care of. So, now he needs to go into a group home. You'll be lucky if he's not raped, or beaten up or doesn't do the beating himself. These children don't know better." I could not hold back my tears envisioning my son being beaten. I was confused and very scared.

The information was more than I could bare but I knew that I needed to let go somehow. The counselor gently passed me a tissue as she began, "Down's children are born with stomach problems, heart problems, vision problems, and many other things." She spoke more softly than the doctor had and I sensed that she was trying to reach me with a pleading tone of voice. "We don't know the severity of his Down's so we don't know what we're in for, not to mention, the government doesn't help financially." The doctor cut in, "Down's children have been known to die young, therefore, he could die from birth to who knows when." Jane spoke up, "If this was your only child, well then, you could place all your attention on him, but you have three small children that you will never be able to spend any time with, because, I'll guarantee you, you will be at hospitals all the time dealing with a sick child." With all the information that was being thrown at me, I just wanted to scream, "Shut up, just shut up," but I just sat with tears rolling down my cheeks, unable to utter a word. I wanted to hide and put my hands over my face. I tried to figure everything out. Angelo cleared his throat and asked, "Would we be able to notice the Down's when he's born?" Jane answered, "When it's a mild case, sometimes it's not noticeable until a few months pass, but when it's severe, sometimes it's noticeable at birth." Angelo sought confirmation for the diagnosis.

Everyone sat quietly and listened to me cry. Finally Jane said, "I have booked you in for tomorrow morning. Come back to genetics at 7:00 AM." As we drove home I wondered what the children had been up to all day. I wondered if Lucy and Gaetano had missed me. My thoughts went to Joseph and I prayed that he did not understand what was going on. I felt as though I had been hit on the head with a large rock. The left side of my temple pounded and I could no longer think. I just wanted to sleep.

The children were happy to see us and I them. We hugged for the longest time and I could not help but think, "At least I did something right with these guys." I looked at my beautiful daughter and asked, "What did you do today?" Lucy said excitedly, "Played." Gaetano's words came pouring out, as though he had held them in for days. "Lucy bad, nonna bottle." I could not quite grasp what he said, but the sound of his voice and his excitement made me smile, "Really, that's great." I was happy for the moment. Joseph was quiet and I did not pressure him to talk. I gave him a hug and said, "I love you more than anything in the world." Nothing else mattered, at that moment, but my husband and my children. I refused to think about tomorrow. I wanted everyone involved to be happy, as we had been before.

- 13 -
We return to the Hospital

The morning seemed like a dejavue. Once again Angelo and I got dressed kissed the children good-bye. Stella said, "Be strong." once again. My mother's eyes were tired and sad. My mother said, "Lina wants to meet you at the hospital." "No Ma, Angelo and I need to be alone. Please thank Lina for her thoughts, but we need to be alone." My mother did not want us to be alone and I knew she would be persistent so I quickly walked away and was relieved that I had managed to avoid more advice.

"What's in your head, share, I need you to share." I asked Angelo, who was deep in thought, as we drove to the hospital. My stare did not allow him the option of not answering me. With his eyes on the road he said, "When I think of him, I picture him as a healthy baby and I can't shake it." My eyes filled with tears and the sorrow I felt for my husband. I wanted Angelo to know that his feelings and thoughts were acknowledged, "I know, I've caught myself thinking that too, but he's not healthy, and we need to realize that. Ang, when we look at our kids we can see they're healthy. I don't even care about the color of his hair or his eyes, I don't even care that his features would be those of a Down's child. My concern is the quality of his life. What would he be in for? What would we be in for?" I stopped talking and hoped Angelo would open up.

For the first time since we received the news, Angelo began to express his feelings, "I remember back in Italy, my parents had some really close friends and they had a Down's child. They used to tell my parents how the kids at school used to tease him and how the brothers used to get into fights with the other kids over it." He continued in a soft voice, "I don't want our kids to go through that. I don't want Luca to go through all the stares and ridicule either." I realized, through Angelo's words, that we were saving our son from a hard life, or were we just saving ourselves from a hard life with him? I wanted so badly to believe our decision was for the best, and hoped God could see that, yet the guilt overpowered all reason in my mind. Both deep in thought we did not say another word for the rest of the drive.

At the hospital we headed straight to the Genetics department. A nurse asked me to change into a gown, and again I headed for the dull gray room. The same doctor that performed the amnio was there, but this time I was unable to be friendly. I needed all my energy for myself and, frankly, I did not care whether I was friendly or not.

The nurse said, "Okay, Antoinette lie down and lift your gown." The doctor walked toward me with a long needle. He tried to be kind but did not say very much. "Okay, now just relax and breathe." He said, before inserting the needle into my vagina. All I could think of was the Lord's Prayer and the Hail Mary, as tears slid into my ears. I repeated the prayers at least three times, concentrating on every word. I hoped and prayed for forgiveness as I felt the tug and the burn inside. The doctor did not take long, but the pain dragged the time out. The nurse rubbed my back and said, "A wheel chair is coming and you'll have a private room."

An unfamiliar woman came and introduced herself, "Hi, I'm Victoria, I'll be helping you through this for the rest of your stay." "Are you feeling anything?" Angelo asked. "Just some cramping, it just feels like cramps from a period. This pain isn't too bad. I thought. Victoria came in to check up on me regularly. Occasionally, she checked my temperature and my blood pressure. She never said a word; she just walked in and did her job.

I began to feel angry and I knew that I could not keep my head down every time she came into the room. I felt as though I was playing the victim and it got on my damn nerves. When Victoria returned, I straightened my back and asked, "Do you think bad of me for this?" She stopped and looked right at me, "I am not here to judge you in any way. I'm only going to help you through this and that's it." As she walked towards the door, she looked back and gave me a comforting smile, "Personally I would have done the same. This world is cruel enough without complications."

Angelo tried to cheer me up. He took all of the children's pictures from his wallet and pinned them on the bulletin board in my room. He tried very hard to be my knight in shining armour. I looked at the pictures and smiled at him with a look of approval, which I knew made him happy. The terrible cramps became stronger and I was nauseous. I went back and forth from the bed to the washroom trying to find a happy medium. Victoria came in and said "Antoinette when you feel the urge to push then just push. This is not a regular pregnancy and you can just push." I began to cry. She came towards me and asked, "Are you in pain?" I mumbled something she could not grasp and she said, "Take a deep breath and say it again." I fumbled once again and through my tears asked, "When he's born will he slowly die in my arms?" She gently placed her hand under my chin and steered my eyes toward her, "No. the doctor stopped his heart beat two hours ago. The needle the doctor gave you at Genetics was for that reason. He's already gone." She brushed my hair back with her hand and walked away. I began to cry even harder and was grateful that I had not really understood the procedure. Had I known what was going on at Genetics, I would probably have been even more hysterical. Now, in my eyes, the deed was done there was no turning back. I almost felt a sense of relief. The pain came stronger and stronger and I knew I could not endure it much longer. I was tired both physically and mentally. When I went to the washroom for the last time I did not realize that the physical pain was coming to an end. I crouched down and the pain subsided. 'Thank God.' I felt a drop and knew it was the baby. I pushed the help button. The cramps had stopped and Victoria came running in. "I felt something drop,"

I said, "Okay. Don't look back. Pick yourself up and go straight to your bed. I did not dare sneak a peek. I was too afraid of what I might see; I did exactly what I was told.

When I returned to the room, Angelo was sitting quietly and patiently with his elbows resting on the bed, his hands pressed together and his forehead leaning on them. I knew he was praying. I stood by the bed with my big white gown dangling off my shoulders and I stared at Angelo. His eyes grew wide and he asked, "Is it done?" I did not have the strength to muster emotion. I nodded and we continued to stare at each other. "It's done." I whispered, and continued to stand there completely numb. My body was tired, my tummy felt hollow, and my soul was defeated. I was a changed woman and Angelo was a changed man, but we were together and strong.

Victoria came in holding the tiniest comforter with blue checkers on it. Inside was Luca. His skin was blue, his eyes were sealed shut and his lips were white. She handed him to me and he was no bigger than my hand. I held him to my chest. My motherly instincts kicked in and I rocked him back and forth. "I'm sorry I'm sorry, I'm sorry, please forgive me." Was all I could say. Angelo had tears in his eyes and he kept rubbing my arm, but he did not have the heart to hold our baby. Stella had given me some holy water in a little bottle and I asked Angelo, to get it for me. We poured some on Luca's head. I prayed to God to take my son home and to accept this blessing. "Dear God please take my son into heaven with you. Please don't punish him for the sins of his parents." I prayed and hoped God was listening. Victoria returned and took him away.

I lay down on my side and fell asleep. It was peaceful and quiet. I did not have to think or make any more decisions; all I had to do was escape from life and sleep. At 9:00 AM a doctor came in with another nurse. He spoke with the nurse but did not say a word to me. He tugged at my tummy to push the embryonic sack out. Victoria and the doctor looked carefully at the sack and I wondered what they were doing. "The IUD didn't come out with the afterbirth. You need to contact you gynecologist and have it removed." The doctor said.

Jane came in; I could not help but notice her bright pink top. I kept looking at her pink top and finally asked, "What's with the bright pink?" She smiled and said, "I was hoping a bright color would cheer you up." "Well it certainly blinded me." I smiled. She was happy to see me smile. "Do you and Angelo want to see the baby one last time?" She asked. I agreed, but as soon as she brought him in, the sadness overwhelmed me again, and the tears followed. I took some pictures of the baby, it gave me a bit of comfort to know that I would always have these pictures and I could see my son whenever I needed to. I held him tightly to my chest and I felt his cold rubbery skin.

Jane pulled the comforter away from his face and said, "Angelo come closer, I want to show you the signs of Down's." Angelo sat up with anticipation. She pointed to the back of the baby's head and said, "See his head, it's larger than a normal baby." Jane looked up at Angelo and continued, "His eyes are closer to each other than normal, and his nose is flat and lower than normal." She carefully rolled the baby to his side and pointed to his ears, "You can see his ears are much lower than they should be." She added, "See the back of his head, as well, is larger than normal. Angelo, his features are so noticeable that I'm pretty sure the baby had severe Down's." She looked at Angelo and asked, "Does this help?" I was happy for Angelo. I knew that all the doubts he had, were relieved with physical evidence before him and he could now move on.

I took a quick shower. Dumping a handful of shampoo into my long blond hair and scrubbed as hard as I could. I grabbed the bar of soap and scrubbed the blood off my legs; the angrier I became, the harder I scrubbed. Finally, I changed into fresh clean clothes and was ready to go home. Jane came in one last time and said, "Here, this is for you." I noticed she was holding the tiny blue checkered comforter and a card. I opened the card and there were Luca's little foot prints. His feet were the size of half my thumb and I just stared at them thinking "what if." But it was too late for what if. Jane hugged me and said, "Time heals all wounds." I looked into her eyes and gave her half a smile. "How does time heal this?" I wondered. As I walked away I thought of Dr. Phil when he said, "Time doesn't heal anything. It's how you choose to handle that time that make's the difference." "I'll call you tomorrow and discuss the baby's burial." Jane called out. I did not look back nor acknowledge her comment. Just a few more minutes and I will be out the doors, and all of this will disappear, like magic, I thought.

At the nurses station, the nurses were either on the phone, shuffling paper or chatting. A nurse looked at me and asked, "May I help you?" "Don't you know who I am? I'm the lady from room 212 who cried all night and aborted her baby. How could you not know who I am?" I thought. I realized at that moment, that if I did not talk about what had happened, no one else would have to know. It no longer mattered and strangers did not care. "Can you please say good-bye to Victoria for me?" I answered. Off we went, empty handed, sad and broken hearted.

We sat silently in the car, buried deep in our own thoughts. I remembered when each one of my children was born, how it was always a celebration. I smiled as I pictured every moment of Joseph's birth. Angelo bought cigars and liquor and passed them, out even to strangers. The happiness was more than any one couple should ever have in a lifetime. We were ecstatic when Gaetano was born; Joseph then had a playmate and a baby brother. Angelo ordered pizza and we feasted like kings at the hospital. We held our children as we tried to chew on the dough, burning our lips on the hot cheese. I laughed over the silliest things, knowing my roommate was right behind the curtain next to me. When Lucy was born, I pictured everyone at the hospital envious of my daughter.

Angelo brought the cappuccino maker from home and we shared coffee with everyone. The nurses came in for a quick espresso. It was so funny, until a security man came in and said it was a fire hazard. He snuck a quick espresso before he told Angelo, "Okay, get it out of here." Angelo was always so proud and he thought everyone else was too. Thinking of my children helped the ride go faster and I smiled to myself for a while until I thought of Luca.

Today was different, there were no funny stories to tell or a baby to hold. There was only my self-doubt, my guilt, and my shame. For the rest of the drive home, I kept thinking, "How do we forgive ourselves? How do we accept and move on?" I looked at Angelo, but there was nothing to talk about. My head was heavy and my eyes wanted to close. I just wanted to get home to my children and pretend this never happened.

- 14 -
Home Again

The children came running to the door. Lucy and Gaetano pushed each other to get to me first. I fell down on my knees and buried my face in both, at the same time. "Come down here and hug your mamma." I told Joseph. I smiled at him as he bent over and wrapped his arms around my neck. I leaned into his ear and said, "I'm going to stay home every day now okay?" The news in Joseph's ears was like sweet candy in his mouth. Stella and my mother waited patiently for their turn. They wanted confirmation that I was alright. We kissed hello, my body began to slow down. I was so drained physically, I needed to sleep. "Anne I'm going to go home." Stella said. I thanked her for her help and went straight upstairs. I lay in bed with my eyes closed and prayed, "Dear God please guide my son into the light." And I fell asleep until the next morning.

I decided to make bacon and eggs for everyone that morning. Angelo came over to the stove, kissed me good morning, and asked, "Are you alright?" I kept my eyes on the pan as the eggs crackled in the oil. I acknowledged his question with a nod and started to cry. My mother who had stayed over, left the room to give us some privacy, Angelo put his hand on my back and in a gentle voice said, "What triggered the cry?" "Choose!...you choose what you think triggered it, and I'll bet you'll win the million dollar prize." Angelo did not dare challenge me, he kissed my cheek and walked away.

The first call of the day rang and rang. I was not going to answer it. I felt comfort in everyone's thoughts, but, at the same time, I wanted to be selfish. I waited for Angelo to answer, after all, I did all the hard work, let him do all the explaining, but I could not stand it any longer. I threw the sponge down and answered the phone myself. It was Angelo's boss. "You and Angelo are very strong people to go through this hardship, and I completely agree and respect your decision." He said and asked, "Is Angelo alright?" "He is trying to be strong for me, but I can see he is really heartbroken." I answered, "I was so sad when Angelo walked into my office with tears and gave me the news." I was taken aback because Angelo usually keeps his business to himself. I had never known him to air his laundry with anyone. I realized at that moment that I had forgotten about Angelo, and I needed to reach out to him.

The phone rang all day, and I answered the calls myself. I somehow found the strength that Angelo now needed from me. Everyone tried to give us words of encouragement and it was well appreciated. At the same time, I really just wanted to tell everyone to leave me alone and let me grieve, this was our time to feel sorry for ourselves. I kept thinking, "I can't allow a song to make me happy. I can't let God see that any little thing throughout the day might make me smile. What if he punishes me for my happiness, when I have taken my son's happiness away?" My faith was with me, but the fear of God was with me even more.

"I am a terrible mother. How in God's name does a mother choose to let her child lay in a cold grave alone." I told myself and felt chilled. I decided to try and make things as right as possible. I sat next to Angelo and held his hand. With tears in my eyes I said in a broken voice, "Do you think we should cremate his little body and keep the ashes here at home?" Angelo's face went white with shock. "Why do you want to do that?" "Ang, I just can't think of him laying out there in the cold alone. He'll be wondering why I abandoned him." I could no longer control my words and the thought of my child far from me was more than I could bare. I cried uncontrollably and my body shook as Angelo held me in his arms. "Let's see what Jane has to say when she calls, then we'll make our decision." Angelo said gently.

Jane's call finally came. "Do you want to take care of your own burial, or do you want the hospital to take care of it?" She asked and explained, "The baby would be cremated and placed with many of the other baby's that died in the last six months." She continued, "The burial will be sometime in April and a letter will be sent to you with all the information you will need." I did not hesitate and said, "Yes, that will be fine. I would like Luca to be buried with the other children." I was truly grateful. I sat at the table and cried, but this time I cried with relief. "Thank God I did something right." I thought and felt in my heart that Luca would not be alone, he would be with all of the other children, and for that I was grateful.

Angelo had gone to work. He found it easier to keep his mind busy and no matter how grief stricken we were, the bills still needed to be paid. I could sense that Angelo did not want to hear about the baby anymore. I felt lonely, and sad, I called my mother, " The baby is going to be buried in April." I said. "If you want, you can bury Luca in my plot." Whenever I visit my father's grave I look at the empty plot next to him and I thank God for the extra years we have had with my mother. My eyes filled with tears. My mother and father had bought adjoining plots to ensure they would be together even in death. Now, she offered to share her burial space for my child. My lower lip began to tremble, I could not speak. I took a deep breath and told her, "Thank you, but he needs to be with the children."

My mother heard me cry and said, "Try to keep your mind busy. You haven't spent much time with the children. You need to get out of the house with them." We began to say good-bye when she said, "You know, Mother Mary gave up her only son to be nailed to the cross to save the world, and you gave up your son to save your other children." "Thank you ma." I could not move, her words were empowering, and I pictured Jesus on the cross. My mother put it all into perspective and I was consoled, knowing the children were safe. All of my children were safe no matter where they were. I wiped my tears, blew my nose, and tried to call the children with a cheery voice. "How about we go to McDonalds?" They jumped up and down. For the first time that week I saw Joseph smile with excitement. Get your shoes on guys." He told the other two. " I felt like their mother again and it felt good. I tried not to think of anything, but giving my children a happy day and a big McDonald's hamburger. I would drown my sorrows in a Big Mac and then some.

The children ran every which way without a care in the world. I watched them laugh and play and socialize with children they did not know. I realized how much I had neglected them and how much I had missed them. Lucy kept coming over and hugging me. Gaetano kept looking over to make sure I was still in my seat. Joseph scurried up and down the slides and I could hear his laughter as he called out for Gaetano. I looked around the room at the mothers playing with their children and talking with friends. I had no desire to speak to anyone and smiling for my children was the best I could do. I kept reminding myself that today was for them, I had plenty of time to cry when we got home.

"Okay guys, mommy has to cook dinner. I want you guys to go into the playroom and play with your toys quietly." They looked tired and I knew they were ready for quiet time. I was happy for my children, but I did not dare feel a sense of contentment myself. As I peeled potatoes at the kitchen sink, I sensed that I was not alone. Joseph came up behind me and stood there. I knew it was Joseph because he stood taller than the other children and he did not tug at my pants. I turned around and went down on one knee. I stared into his beautiful eyes and he seemed very serious. I realized this was not a mere visit. I wanted Joseph to know that he had my undivided attention. I put my hands on his shoulders, and said, "What's up baby?" Without a moments hesitation he said, "Today was a good day!" I smiled "Ya, did you have fun at McDonald's?" He continued to stare into my eyes, and with the softest voice said, "No, because you didn't cry today."

I pulled Joseph towards me and held him as tight as I could. I tried not to cry so that he would not feel me tremble.

Months ago when I was sick with a high fever, I spent the day sleeping off and on. I tried to take care of the children, but I was very weak and got off the sofa only when I had no choice. Joseph came to me and said, "Here mommy." He was holding a bottle of Tylenol in one hand and a plastic cup of water in the other. As sick as I was, I could not help but laugh, I was so surprised. I was about to thank him when he said, "I couldn't open the bottle." "You really are the best kid in the world." I dragged myself off of the sofa and thought, "I better see what they want to eat." I walked into the kitchen and saw the container of butter and a loaf of bread on the floor. Joseph followed me into the kitchen and said, "I made the kids butter sandwiches for lunch." I sat on the floor, pulled Joseph into my arms, and hugged him. "Thank you for being my son." I realized at that moment that Joseph was a kind person with a big heart.

I had always known Joseph was mature for his age and he proved it time and again. "When I was sick that day he knew what pills would make me better. Now he's trying to heal me mentally." I thought and all my thoughts were of him. Joseph gently pulled himself from my grip and walked away. I became angry with myself. I knew Joseph was sensitive. I knew he picked up on everything. I knew he was hurting. I knew, I knew, I knew.

I could not believe how much pain my child was in. "How could I have done this to him? How could I have hurt him like this?" My mother's face flashed through my mind and I thought of her words. "You gave up your son to save your other children." I leaned against the sink and said to myself. "Okay. This is it, from now on I will only allow myself to cry when the children cannot hear me." Luca's death was not in vain. In the short time I held Luca in my arms, he taught me to appreciate my children. He made me realize that God blessed me with motherhood and that I must live up to the title. I would not allow my days to be all about me any longer. My pain was mine and mine alone.

"Did Jane call today?" Angelo asked when he came home. "Yes." I answered. "I don't want anyone coming to the burial." He said in a stern tone of voice. I knew to leave well enough alone, but my curiosity got the better of me. "Okay, but why?" He stared at the television for a couple of seconds, "We don't need a big production. I just don't want anyone there." He said and raised the volume, letting me know the conversation was over. I knew he was in pain and decided to honor his wishes.

My days filled with phony smiles and my nights were riddled with guilt and remorse. I cried every night in bed; I was desperate to protect my children from my tears. I held my pillow tightly around my face and with each wail the heat from my breath suffocated me. My prayers never altered and I begged my father to take care of Luca. "Please pappa, let me know if you have the baby." I would beg, "Pappa, please guide him to you. He will be scared alone." Finally, I would threaten, "Pappa if you don't give me a sign I will stop praying to you." My pleading was desperate and I would have said anything for a sign from the heavens.

I begged for all the calls to stop and when they finally slowed down, I was angry that everyone had moved on. My brother Guy and his wife Mary invited us for dinner. Although I spoke to Mary everyday, we had not seen each other since that day. At dinner, I could not stop talking about my faith. I spoke of God's prayers and tried to analyze God's words. Mary never once interrupted me and said, "I'm happy you didn't lose your faith. Ant, I have never seen you so broken." She never once tried to change the topic. I told her about Luca's burial and she said, "Ant, whatever you guys want, we will do."

Guy said "Ant, I would have done the same thing, now get over it." I was so surprised by what he said that I could not help but laugh. It was a bittersweet evening. Angelo and I really needed a break, yet I felt guilty for having a bit of fun. The children had a wonderful time with their cousins and they slept all the way home.

- 15 -
The Nursery

Lucy and Gaetano seemed to return to their routine, but Joseph was still very reserved. I decided that he deserved some kind of explanation. One day as I was driving with the children, I thought it was a good time. But how much did they know? How much have they understood? I shut off the radio and asked, "Hey guys, can we talk about the baby that was in mommy's tummy?" I looked in the rear view mirror. I had everyone's attention. "Did you know the baby in mommy's tummy was sick?' Joseph answered, "Ya." Gaetano answered the same. "Well Jesus decided he needed to take the baby back and fix him," I continued. "Is Jesus going to give him back when he's fixed?" Joseph asked. "No baby, mommy is too old to carry him in my stomach again, but maybe Jesus will give him to another family when he is better." I was at a red light and looked into the mirror. Gaetano's eyes widened and he sat up in his chair "Did an alien take the baby?" he asked. I chuckled and said, "Ya, I guess so." It was very quiet in the van and I was not sure what more to say. Then Joseph said, "If I get sick is God gonna take me too?" I choked back my tears, and pulled to the side of the road. "No Joseph, if you get sick the doctor will fix you and let you stay with me. The reason why Jesus had to take him back was because he was in my tummy and the doctor's couldn't reach him." I asked him if he understood, and he just said, "Ya." Lucy was fast asleep. The children never talked about it again.

I tossed and turned all night dreaming of the nursery. I was painting the room in sky blue, but as the paint dried the color changed to dark purple. I became annoyed and frantically painted the walls over and over again. When I awoken I felt nervous and anxious. "I need to box up the nursery, that's what I need to do today!" I grabbed a handful of garbage bags and was excited to keep my hands and mind busy. I started with the baby clothes. I picked up a pair of newborn pajamas and held it to my face. I could smell the scent of baby powder and the softness felt good against my cheek. I tried to picture the boys in the pajamas but my thoughts always returned to Luca. My eyes filled with tears, as I emptied the drawers, filled the garbage bags, and discarded my past.

I tried to concentrate on the task, but I kept thinking of nursery rhymes. I started to box up the baby powders, wipes, and face clothes. I reached into the back of the change table and pulled out a brand new bag of diapers. I sat on the rocking chair and thought, "I never got to use these." I sat for a while but I had no desire to cry. "Mamma called the doctor and the doctor said, no more monkeys jumping on the bed." I repeated the nursery rhyme over and over in my mind. I became agitated and annoyed. I grabbed a screwdriver and took the change table apart. Then, I gently took the basinet apart tucking it into the back of the empty closet. "Mamma called the doctor, and the doctor said." Finally I looked at the crib, my voice cracked "No more monkeys jumping on the bed." I began to cry, "Why God, why did you choose me?" I walked over to the crib and began to tear the bedding off and threw it to the floor. I was angry with myself. I wanted my son to sleep in a warm crib not in a grave. My cries became a screeching sound as I fell to the floor holding onto the bars of the white lacquer crib.

I thought of my first baby shower and the big box the crib came in. When the guests had all gone, my sisters decided to set the crib up before they left. Lina, Pina, Maria, Stella, Tracey, my mother, Angelo and me gathered into the nursery. I was not surprised at their intentions, but Angelo had no idea what to expect. "Stand back ladies and watch the master at work." Angelo thought he would be the brain behind the project, but, honestly, he was not given the chance. "Angelo get out of our way." My sister's said. Everyone grabbed a piece from the box and it was set up in less than an hour. When the last piece was in place I looked at Angelo and began to laugh. I was used to my sisters ways. My father had taught us how to use hammers, nails, screws, screwdrivers, and other tools that he owned. Angelo, on the other hand, was impressed.

I thought about Joseph in his crib. He did not sleep in it very much. He was my firstborn and I could not part from him, so most nights he slept in our bed and remained in our bed until, well, forever. When we passed the crib down to Gaetano I was grateful it was still brand new. Gaetano never really cried when it was bedtime and slept quietly through the night, until he figured out that Joseph slept in our bed. When he was about eight months old, he moved in with us as well, and it became a little tight. Lucy too, slept in the same crib and it was still fairly new. She needed to be rocked before she could be put down in the crib but that never bothered me and once she fell asleep it was easy sailing. Then she decided she wanted in on the good deal the boys had. So I would let them all start off in our bed and when they fell asleep, Angelo and I took them to their rooms.

As I remained on the floor, I could not allow myself to fall in love with my memories of the crib and the children. There were no memories of Luca and that was entirely my fault. Guilt went through me like a knife and I had to get out of the room. I closed the door behind me and ran to the washroom. I washed my face and swore I would never enter the nursery again until Angelo took the crib apart. I did not enter the room for months and kept telling Angelo that I wanted to sell the house. I felt guilty that we had such a big home and could not fill it as we had intended. Angelo ignored my pleas and one Saturday morning he turned the room into a "Computer room." It no longer looked like a nursery and my need to move out eventually subsided.

- 16 -
Preparing for a Burial

The children enjoyed our morning walks. We headed away from the mailbox and would pick up the mail on our way home. I started taking longer routes knowing that one day there would be a letter from Jane advising me about the funeral. My morning walks became stressful, and the further away from the mailbox I walked, strangely enough, the faster I walked to get to it. I did not want to read about the plans for my son's burial, and yet I wanted it to be over. Then the day came. As I walked faster toward the mailbox my breath became heavier, the heat poured into my face, but that was nothing compared to the pounding in my chest just before I reached my destination. I stood in front of the mailbox with the keys in my hand and stared at the white envelope addressed to Angelo and me. I read the hospital's logo over and over, wondering what was inside. I could not wait I sat down at the edge of the sidewalk and tore the envelope open. I took a deep breath and muttered, "Dear God here we go with the next phase to deal with." The letter, typed on the hospital letterhead, was dated March 2004. It seemed strange that there wasn't an actual date on it. The letters were in blue and I thought, "That's a nice touch, it brightens up the paper." With great anticipation I read.

> *Dear Friends,*
>
> *We want to convey our understanding of the loss of your child. Losing a life which was just beginning is an especially difficult loss to bear, for in saying goodbye to this small person.*

I stopped for a moment to grab a tissue from the bottom of the stroller. The children were playing and I gave them some cookies hoping that would keep them busy for a couple of minutes. I wanted to concentrate on every word, even though I knew that I would read the letter a dozen more times.

> *"We also acknowledge all of the unfulfilled hopes and dreams you cherished. To assist in the healing of those wounded places in your heart, we have planned a special service of remembrance, as outlined in the release form you signed when you were in the hospital. You, and as many others as you would like to bring, are invited to a Service of Remembering and Healing to acknowledge the life and love you will always have for your little one.*
>
> *When: Saturday April 24, 2004 (rain or shine)*

Where: High hills Memorial Gardens

Time: 11:00 am – the service will be approximately ½ hour long.

We will meet at the Garden of Angel's; Parking is available on the edge of the road. We will meet together at the graveside. You'll see the green grass set up and cemetery staff will be able to assist you if you have any difficulties with the directions.

Our time together will give you the opportunity to share with other families who understand your grief, to remember your child, and to say a special goodbye in a multi faith environment. If you would like to bring flowers to leave at the graveside, please feel free to do so. You may also bring one very tiny momento to be placed in the grave, if so desired. Please understand that it must be very small."

My mind went into overdrive. I wanted to put something very special in Luca's grave. It had to be something between him and me, something I could also have around, at all times to feel him close. I could not put a toy in, that would be too big. I needed to find that perfect something, but what?

Angelo read the letter, he did not say a word. He passed the letter back to me and walked away. He was distraught; his big bright happy eyes were dim, sad, and tired. His voice lost its sparkle and I could sense that he did not want to deal with the funeral. I was sad for him. Once again my heart knocked at my chest reminding me that we were both broken. "That's it, a broken heart, oh my God, that's it. I'll put half in his grave and half will remain on my necklace." I was relieved knowing that my son would receive his one and only gift from mommy and daddy.

I called Stella, "Do you know where I can buy a gold heart?" I explained what it was for, hoping she would take on the task of finding it. "I have a great jeweler who will have it for sure." Stella answered, "Great!" I did not have the strength to do it myself and was relieved she had the time. "When do you need it by?" "I have to have it by April 24th. If you can't get it to me, I'll find a day to drive over to your place and pick it up." "Don't worry, I'll come up for a visit sometime next week and get it to you." She said happily.

I tried not to think about it for the next few days but I kept fantasizing about the funeral. I pictured myself placing the gold heart in the urn. "I wonder what I'll say. I wonder what others will put." Stella knocked on my door and I was excited to see what she had chosen. It was an 18 karat gold heart with diamonds all around it and the words "Together Forever." I hugged her, "Stella, it's exactly what I wanted, it's beautiful." "I'm glad you're happy. I have one more thing." She said and opened a tiny box, she held in her hands. It was a gold baptismal medallion with the Mother Mary holding a baby, and on its back the word "Baptism." I took it gently out of the box and held it in the palm of my hand. The gold was yellow and shiny, and it was beautiful. As I stared at it Stella said, "I wanted this to be placed in his grave as well." Angelo and I knew Stella would have been a great godmother to Luca, and as bitter sweet as this moment was, I knew she was the right choice.

I waited at the counter at the photo lab to receive the pictures I had taken of Luca. My stomach became heavy and I felt nauseous. I kept thinking the clerk would hand me the envelope and say something really hurtful. I was embarrassed and I just wanted to pay and run out. At home I stared at Angelo sitting in the family room and said, "I have the pictures of the baby." He did not look up, nor did he stop watching television. He nodded and bit his lower lip. I waited by the sofa but after a few moments I decided no to push the issue. I never brought it up again, neither did Angelo. I placed the pictures carefully in a small photo album to preserve the only pictures I would ever have of Luca. I rubbed my fingers over each picture trying to remember what he felt like, how he smelled. I held back my tears and hid the photo album in his green keepsake box. Every night, for months, I took the pictures out and held them close to me. I took comfort in them knowing I could see Luca and pray to him. "Please forgive me, my baby. Sleep well." I ended my prayer with, "Daddy, I hope you have him safe in your arms."

- 17 -
A Family Feud

Every day felt the same to me. My mind remained on the day of the burial. I stole moments throughout the day to cry privately without the children knowing. Everyone's lives moved on, and we were close to the end of March. Birthdays were coming up on Angelo's side of the family and they were to be celebrated. Angelo's parents invited family members over to their house. This was the first time I would see his side of the family since the abortion and I was very nervous. I was not in a festive mood, but I tried to be polite. Angelo and I met relatives who had backed us in our decisions and relatives who did not. Every look I received, I took personally, and thought, "Are they trying to stare me down?"

I decided to approach the one person whose comments had been the most hurtful "Sue, Do you think you could come outside with me for a moment?" I asked. I was calm and did not want to be confrontational. "Even though I didn't appreciate your comment about raising my son, I'm not going to be mad at you, I just want to put it aside and move on." I began. "Why, is Angelo mad at me?" Sue asked. "Well, he wasn't thrilled with your comment, but he just wants to forget about it too." Sue and I agreed to put the past behind us and move on, or so I thought.

After dinner the children scattered in the family room. Sue confronted Angelo, "Are you mad that I offered to raise the baby?" Everyone stopped what they were doing to listen I had dirty dishes in my hands but I stopped and placed them on the table. "Your comment was stupid, you had no reason to say that." Angelo answered. Others at the table said, "This topic is too delicate. Just drop it." "I thought this was settled." I questioned Sue. She ignored me completely and everyone began to speak at the same time. I knew by Sue's tone of voice that she wanted Angelo to fulfill her selfish needs and comfort her. I was angry and thought, "As usual no regard for what we've been through. It's always about her."

"Everyone just stop it. There is no need to get into this conversation, just stop!" I said. Sue's sister Kate stood up and said, "Oh, boo hoo, I have no pity for you, that baby was four months old and you killed him. You're a baby killer." No sooner did she finish her devilish words, Angelo was already at the other end of the table. He faced her and said, "Get out of this house." His voice was so loud that it caught everyone's attention. They all began screaming at each other. Angelo began to fight with Kate's husband and everyone tried to break it up. Angelo's parents kicked everyone out to keep us apart. We struggled to get our coats and round up our children. I was shaken. Sue shouted at me, "I never want to see you again, and I'm glad my sister said it... you are a baby killer."

Sue continued looking directly at me, "I hope God punishes you for what you have done. You deserve to go to hell." We made our way to the van. I tried to buckle the children in as fast as I could but my hands trembled and I fumbled. Finally we drove away. I kept touching my neck, feeling the bump that grew larger by the minute. I wiped away the blood, but the throbbing would not stop. Angelo kept saying, "They went too far." Joseph kept asking, "Mommy what happened?" I didn't answer.

I went to the doctor a couple of days later. My neck was still red and the vein was purple and stuck out quite a bit. "A nerve was hit. It will take a while before it heals." The doctor said. But the reality was that the physical would not hurt nearly as much as the emotional pain and doubt we felt. After that day Angelo and me began to doubt ourselves. We thought of the terrible words that were said to us. I wondered if we were doomed for judgment day and I became afraid. "Do you think God really will punish us?" I asked Angelo. Angelo replied in a stern voice, "Don't listen to anything they said." he hesitated, and then added, "I don't know, I hope not."

The family feud stayed with me every moment of the day. I felt lost with God and my energy for prayers was at its lowest; I just wanted to lay in bed all the time, but my thoughts would not allow me to asleep. I became paranoid for my children. I prayed, " God are you going to punish me through my kids?" I kept asking, "God was that fight a sign from you?" The fear and shame became too much to handle as the days passed. I finally saw the doctor and began to cry uncontrollably. "You have nothing to be ashamed of." He said. "I'm going to prescribe some anti-depressants. It will help you through the days with your depression." The pills gave me some energy to get through the day, but I became extremely shaky and my sisters were concerned.

Maria and Stella came over during the week. "What brought on this depression?" Maria asked. I could not hold it in any longer and I cried. I explained in detail everything said the night of the fight. "Since then I can't stop thinking God's going to punish us." I hoped that Maria would reassure me that I was not going to be punished and that God has nothing to forgive. "They have no right to cast a stone. They have no idea what God is thinking or what his plans are. Maybe they better worry about God's plan for them." Stella said. As I wiped away my tears I tried to calm down. Stella continued, "They were just trying to be as mean as they could. God will punish them in his own time." "How will I know if God does?" I asked. Stella laughed and said, " When God does punish them, you may not be a witness to the fact, but their day will come. God doesn't need your approval for whatever plans he has for others." I thought about Stella's words and said, "I don't want anyone to be punished. I just want them to see how mean and hurtful they are."

- 18 -
Luca's Funeral

The house was quiet. The children were taking a nap and Joseph was at school. I was shaky from the pills and felt sad. I wanted our lives to be happy again, but how could I do that if I did not know the meaning of happiness anymore. I sat on my bed staring at myself in the mirror on my vanity table. I could not stop staring and I could not believe how much I had changed. I stood up and threw my nightgown over the mirror. I could not stand to see the reflection of the person that was supposed to be me. I decided to have a heart to heart with God, Suora Anna Maria Rosa, Mother Mary and, of course, my father. I held my hands together and said, "I will never know why you chose Angelo and me to carry this burden. I hope you all can be proud of the fact that we did our best to be strong and handle it the best way that we knew. Now you've got us doubting every decision and every step we've taken. I'm scared and I'm sad and, most of all, I'm ashamed." I placed my face in my hands and began to cry. "Please guide me through our faith because I'm really losing it. I don't know how much more I can take. Please help me. Please. Daddy please, give me a sign let me know you have him. I'm still waiting for your sign." I was shaky and I knew it was one of the side effects of the pills. I flushed the pills down the toilet and convinced myself, "Come on Ant, your stronger than those pills."

Saturday April 24, 2004. My friend Carol offered to take care of the children while Angelo and I went to the service. I kissed the children, "I won't be gone long." They were excited to have their friends over, and I knew they were not worried about where we were going. I dreaded the drive ahead of us. It gave Angelo and me more time to dwell on the entire situation and we would drive ourselves crazier. Angelo bit his lower lip and I stared out the window, holding the medallion and the heart in a little red box. The day was very windy, and the sun was nowhere to be found. I stared at the clouds and tried to picture what the service would be like. All I could imagine were strangers wearing black, but worse, I kept picturing my son. I knew he was cremated, but I kept picturing him in a casket wearing a beautiful white baptismal gown. He seemed so peaceful, and I thought, "What the hell have I done?" Tears began to fall down my face and the faster I wiped them the harder and faster they fell. Angelo rubbed his hand gently on my head, as though he knew what I was thinking. I could not hold it in anymore, "I can't believe we're going through this." I cried.

Angelo struggled to figure out the location on the map. It took us a while but we finally saw many cars and strangers all huddled around three women. I looked around and spotted Jane. She waved, and pointed to a parking spot. Angelo took my hand and we locked eyes. "Ready?" "Ya, you?" Angelo smiled and we walked towards the group.

He stood behind me and placed his hands on my shoulders. I was cold and shivers crawled up and down my arms. The women introduced themselves as reverends.

"Good morning everyone. As I was getting ready this morning I had the radio on, and a song from Sara McLaughlin came on. I listened to the words and found them to be appropriate for this day. Her song said, 'in the arms of an Angel far away from here, in the arms of an Angel may you find some comfort here?' Everyone in the crowd began to cry and I struggled to find a tissue in my purse. The words were powerful and I prayed Luca was in the arms of an Angel. As I stood in the cold, I noticed a familiar face. It was the Asian woman from the clinic. She looked at me and we exchanged a nod. In some strange way, I felt that my nod let her know I was there for her. The Minister began the service.

"For parents gathered here as they mourn the loss of their child, we pray that God will continue to strengthen and heal them through our compassion and love. We pray, God of compassion, hear our prayer. God of compassion, in whom all life and death find meaning, we bless you at all times, especially when we have need of your consolation. These parents entrust to your care a life conceived in love. May your blessing come upon them now. Remove all anxiety from their minds and strengthen their love so they may have peace in their hearts and homes." She read through the list of children and blessed them, then she said "Naming and entrusting to God's Embrace, baby of Antoinette and Angelo and everyone answered "We entrust you to God's embrace."

As the minister continued to read the names of the children, Angelo shook my shoulder and whispered in my ear, "Ant look down." I turned to him and asked, "What?" he said, "I'm really serious. Look down." I turned and looked down. I was standing on a gold plaque. Angelo stepped back and pulled me off the plaque so I could see it in front of me. Shivers flew across my shoulders and down my back. The plaque read "Baby born of Cosenza." I knew it was a sign from my father letting me know he had Luca with him. I looked at Angelo and, with my lower lip quivering, I said, "Oh my God that's my maiden name." Even though I knew it was obviously another child's grave, I knew it was a sign from my father. What were the odds that I would be standing on it? I looked up at the sky, and said, "Thank you daddy, Thank you."

I was at peace and relieved for a moment. Then I heard the minister blessing us. She picked up a red satin pouch and inside it was the urn. She placed it into a hole in the ground and my heart sank. The ground looked dark, damp, and cold. She completed the service saying, "O god, by whose mercy these little ones find rest, and as we leave this place, we ask you to send your holy Angel to watch over this grave." She continued, "We send with each of you, a tree, a gift as life is a gift. A gift for you to plant in remembrance of the life that you shared with your child, and as a sign that hope and life endure. Go now in God's love and peace. Amen"

People began walking to the grave, one at a time, with their families. Some threw dirt in and I wondered what the significance of that was. I saw a woman throw a letter in and I could imagine a mother's words to her child. Then it was our turn. Angelo and I walked up to the grave I knelt down on my knees and gently put my gift in. Through my tears I said, "Luca hold on to the heart, and one day we will put our hearts together, and our hearts will become one again. This is one promise I will carry to my own grave." Angelo leaned over me and pulled me away so others could have their turn. As I rose I whispered, "I'm sorry, please forgive me." I stood tall, looking at the urn, and said, "I love you, Good-bye."

Jane handed me a little remembrance tree and gave me a big hug. "How are you doing?" she asked. "I'm okay, this was such a difficult day." Jane rubbed my back, and I said, "Can you come to the van with me for a minute?" We walked arm in arm, and I was excited to give her a gift to let her know how much I appreciated her. Jane was very pleased. I gave her a small wooden statue of the Angel of healing. "I'm so grateful for your help, most of all your strength." Jane's eyes teared up and she said, "You have such a beautiful family. Now go home and move on with your lives. Take care of your three beautiful children." We hugged and Jane said, "I will cherish my Angel forever."

As we left the cemetery I asked Angelo, "Can you bring me back in the next couple of weeks so I can get a picture of the tombstone?" "Ok, I'll bring you back just once for your picture but I'm never coming back after that." I was sad, knowing Angelo wanted to forget about our son. Hearing his words forced me to challenge him and I said, "Why wouldn't you want to come back? Ang, this is a part of our lives now and I'm not just going to abandon him or pretend this never happened." Angelo continued driving, never once making eye contact and said, "Ant, what if we did keep him, maybe we would have been okay." I sensed the pain and guilt in his voice and answered, "It's too late to second guess ourselves. What we need to do now is to forgive ourselves. That's the hard part." It started to rain and I wanted to believe that the Angels felt our pain and were crying with us.

- 19 -
A New Normal

We tried to return to normal. It was never going to be the normal we once knew but I was the wife and mother of the family and I needed to create a fresh new normal, if not for myself then for Angelo and the children. The children went back to their routine and Angelo worked harder than ever, and me, well, not an hour passed that I did not think about Luca. I prayed a lot, but mostly to ask for forgiveness, and I constantly fed my sorrows with plenty of food. I knew I was overeating. I felt sick, but I could not stop and it reminded me of my years in high school.

My years in high school were the hardest years for me. I never felt pretty because of my weight, and that would make me eat even more. Once in grade 10 I was sitting on the bleachers with a bunch of friends and we talked about the perfect woman. One of the boys stood up. Edgar was tall, with long silky black hair. He was the most popular boy in school, and he knew it. Edgar said laughing, "The perfect woman for me would be Antoinette's face on Joanne's slender body." I looked at my friend Joanne, and she did not look very happy. We were the same height but she was half my size. Everyone agreed I had the perfect face, but it was not a compliment. It was hurtful to both Joanne and me. I went home and ate away the pain.

Once, in grade 12, I was eating a plate of pasta and my sister Maria asked, "Do you really have to eat all that?" I nodded in reply. "That's okay, we'll just have to find you a fat husband." Her words kept me awake the entire night and the next day I went on a diet. I worked out every evening and within seven months I was slim enough to wear a size 9. I was seven sizes smaller and I felt great.

When I finished reminiscing about my days in high school I found other reasons to continue to eat, like the family feud. The family feud lingered in my mind throughout the days. Although Angelo and I tried not to discuss it much, I knew we both dwelled on the situation often. Angelo became quieter with every passing day and I saw the hurt in his eyes. "Is anything on your mind?" I asked. "I never expected my family to be so unkind. I honestly thought someone would have called by now to apologize." I tried my hardest not to make mean comments about them, because I loved Angelo enough to spare his feelings. "Ang, it's just you and me. No one else matters." I said, but I wanted to say, "How could family do something so mean and not even feel remorse?" I did not share my feelings with Angelo, but I spent many nights thinking of how God would punish them. I wanted everyone to understand our pain, but, on the other hand, I felt relieved that I did not have to face Sue and Kate anymore.

There were days I was angry with myself for obsessing about them as often as I did. Once on the Dr. Phil show, he said, "Don't give someone that kind of power over you." It was so powerful. I ran to get a pen and paper and wrote down his words. I repeated his words to myself until they became a matter of fact, and I decided that their cruelty was not about me but part of their own issues. I understood that I did not need to carry their problems. Angelo and I knew we had to move on with our lives, having survived through the guilt of the abortion. We made it past the funeral as well, and now we needed to mend our souls. We tried not to talk about the family feud or the baby very often.

In the evenings before they fell asleep, ever since Joseph was small, I told the children the story of Jacomino, Pasqualino and their sister Laduika, fictional siblings that lived in Italy. I would use slang phrases my parents had used with their Italian accents. Joseph loved these stories. The story for the evening would reflect on something that had happened during the day. Eventually Jacomino and Pasqualino became family and the children grew to love them.

When Gaetano grew a little older he would ask for a Jacomino Pasqualino story. One evening he asked, "Is Jacomino and Pasqualino our cousins?" I smiled and said, "Kind of." Joseph then asked, "When are we going to visit them?" I lay Joseph and Gaetano in bed and explained, "Well, they are not real, they're just real in our heads and in our hearts." They both looked disappointed. "I have a wonderful story about best friends who had never met Jacomino and Pasqualino but only knew them from letters."

I told the children all about the wonderful secrets they wrote and how their fictional cousins would write back. At the end of the story Joseph and Gaetano said, "We want to write Jacomino and Pasqualino a letter too. A real letter that we can mail." They were so excited, Joseph jumped out of his neatly tucked comforter and began to explain what he wanted to write in the letter. Gaetano followed Joseph's lead and repeated Joseph's every word. I said, "Okay, but for now you both need to sleep. I will help Lucy write a letter to Laduika too."

The boys had finally settled down and Lucy had already fallen asleep. It was my time to wind down and I looked forward to an espresso and spending time with Angelo. I lay next to Angelo staring at the television, but my mind was elsewhere. "I'm going to call Dr. Slater in the morning and schedule to have my tubes tied." Angelo did not move a muscle, nor did he say much for a while. "Would you consider trying one more time?" he asked. I was very surprised. Having another baby never entered my mind. I tried to smile, but a sick feeling came over me and my face felt really hot. There was no way I was ever going to chance it again. "Angelo I hope God has forgiven us for our decisions, and I pray nothing else this devastating ever happens to us again, but I know God won't forgive us a second time." "I would like to try again but I don't want you to go through any more" he said. "Once forgiven twice forgotten." I said sternly. I felt annoyed at him and walked away. I was very angry. "What the hell is he thinking? Did he forget already the hell we have been through?" I was angry at Angelo's request, yet I felt guilty that I could not give him the fourth child he really wanted. I then reverted back to the anger, it was easier to deal with. With my face in my pillow I cried away the evening.

Dr. Slater performed the surgery to tie my tubes. I was brought into my semi private room and woke up in excruciating pain. I pushed the morphine button but it did not help much. "Well, maybe I deserve all this pain." I thought. Dr. Slater came in and said, "Antoinette, we had to give you a bikini c-section. We couldn't poke through the mesh, that thing is like cement." He continued, "You will be able to leave in a few days." "Did you get the IUD out?" I asked. He replied with a smile, "Yes, it was buried deep inside the uterus." Angelo walked in with the children and I could tell he was overwhelmed. I hugged the children and chuckled noticing their clothes. "Ang, the kids look so cute. You color coordinated their clothes." Angelo was proud and said, "My kids need to look good."

I pointed down to Gaetano's shoes and said, "Those runners are Joseph's. They're too big for Gaetano." Angelo laughed, "I know. I couldn't find his." I was proud of my domesticated husband but knew he needed me to come home soon. My hospital visit was restful and gave me time to think. I felt sad knowing I would not have any more babies around the house but I did not want to deal with that. I just wanted to get well enough to go home before Easter.

- 20 -
A Road Trip

The months passed and we headed into the summer. My c-
section healed and I did not cry as often. Phone calls were
not always about the tragedy, but, somehow or someway,
I would find the opportunity to bring it up. Even if the
subject did not last very long, I still found a reason to talk
about it. I felt so different inside. There was a constant
emptiness that I did not know how to fill. My shoulders
felt heavy with the burden of sadness and guilt that I
refused to release.

Lucy began to speak more freely and she asked a lot of
questions. We were sitting at the kitchen table having
fun with arts and crafts. Lucy looked over at me and said,
"Mommy is nonno Joe in heaven?" she was referring to
my father. I was surprised she brought him up and I said,
"Yes, nonno Joe is in heaven." She started to color and

asked, "He's in heaven with the baby right?" The glue fell out of my hand. I lifted her onto my lap and said, "Lucy, what baby?" "Nonno Joe's baby!" She answered. I could not speak. I placed her back in her seat and ran to the washroom. Tears filled my eyes and I said, "Thanks dad, thanks for that." A few weeks later, I asked Lucy about the baby with nonno Joe, and she seemed confused. She did not remember what she had said.

In July, Angelo decided that we needed a vacation. " My holidays begin today. Pack a couple of bags and let's go." "Angelo we can't just up and leave." I said, "Ant I'm leaving by 3:00 PM today. Be packed or I'm leaving without you." I started to laugh "What the hell, maybe this is what we need." I took a bag out of the closet and started packing two weeks worth of clothes for each child. When I tried to fit all the clothes in the one luggage it was too much and I could not get it closed. So I packed one week's worth for each child and that worked better. "It's just as well, if I pack enough clothes for everyone, Angelo won't let me buy any along the way." I quietly chuckled to myself.

We got in the van and the children were beyond excitement. Gaetano was now out of diapers and I would chuckle every time I looked at him in a pair of shorts because he had such a tiny bum. I never realized how skinny he really was. He looked like a little boy now. He had the longest lashes and everyone always commented on them, and his blond hair was always so thick that when it grew a little, his face would be lost. Lucy was now in pull-ups. She was completely determined to follow in Gaetano's footsteps. As soon as Lucy saw Gaetano sitting on the potty, she was anxious to copy him. I tried to convince her to keep her diapers on for a little while longer, but she refused to have anything to do with them. I put her on the potty and she never had an accident. She seemed so tiny to be out of diapers, with her curly blond hair and she was so chubby and cute with her big brown eyes. People told me she looked exactly like Drew Barrymore.

Angelo wanted Lucy in pull-ups at all times during the trip. "I don't want to keep stopping every hour." He filled the tank with gas, paid the bill and walked back to the van holding a map. He opened it up and said, "So which way should we go?" His face was rosy and he looked excited, staring at me in anticipation. I smiled and said "Let's hit the West coast, since we've already done the East coast." We started driving away and I was very excited. I told the children where we were going and they started to ask a million questions.

We drove to Thunder Bay, where we stopped to see the statue of Terry Fox. I told Angelo that I wanted to go to Shania Twain's town, but he laughed and said, "When she visits us, we'll visit her." We drove about six hours on the first day; the children began to get frustrated and started bickering with each other, so we stopped for food. We decided to go to grocery stores for food, to save a little money. When we arrived at the motel, we put on our bathing suits and ran to the indoor pool. The children were so happy, the boys must have gone down the water slide a million times. I sat in the shallow end, so Lucy could splash around while I kept an eye on Angelo and the boys.

Every once in a while I thought of the baby; that we could have taken this trip the following year as a family of six. He could have come in the water with us, or maybe Lucy and I would have stayed back in the room while he slept. Then I thought, no we would probably be at a hospital in Toronto getting some tests or diagnosis done for him and our children would be at home with a baby sitter. I kept telling myself to face the reality of what would have been had we kept him, but no matter how much I tried to reason with myself, it did not change my feelings of guilt and shame. I felt the urge to call one of my sisters and tell them about our bitter sweet vacation, but for the next couple of weeks I did not have time to be on the phone and there was nobody to cry to.

We drove day after day, pointing to all the beautiful mountains and scenery. The mountains came alive with vegetation and wild animals peered out every once in a while. Joseph kept asking, "When are we going to see a bear family cross our path?" "Oh, I don't know. We'll just have to keep searching." I answered. We drove to Banff, Alberta, to the glaciers and Angelo and the boys walked up a portion of the mountain. It was like winter on the mountains and the cold cut through my skin and went straight into my bones. I had no interest in following the boys. "Lucy is too small, I'll stay back with her." People had coats and gloves on while Angelo wore only jeans and runners. The boys had pants on but no coat, so they grabbed beach towels and off they went. I saw the wind tug at their towels and I prayed they would not get sick. They did not go for long, it was much too cold for them to continue. They got down to the bottom and ran to the van. Joseph kept saying, "I'm freezing let me in the van." We spent the days sight seeing and made it our mission to check into motels with water slides.

I took pictures everywhere, including the potty moments, when we pulled off to the side of the highway and I took out our little white potty. The children would sit down and do their business while huge trucks passed by. We went all the way to Calgary, for the Calgary stampede, where the only songs on the radio were country. We found a town called Drumheller; where dinosaurs had been excavated and they built a big museum for tourists with a giant dinosaur. We climbed hundreds of stairs and ended up at the dinosaur's mouth and looked at the scenery. It was really cool and the children could not stop talking about it. It was a very good day, a happy day, a normal day. From there we drove to Edmonton and went to the biggest mall I had ever seen. We were there for hours and did not see the entire mall.

I was determined to see an Indian Pow Wow, so at every information booth we went to, I asked, but no one knew of any happening soon. We were on the second week of our travels and I was very quiet all morning. I felt a sadness come over me and I knew exactly why. Angelo wanted to get on the road early that morning and I felt very teary eyed. Today would have been the day of my fourth child's birth. "Do you know what today is?" I asked Angelo. He reached over, squeezed my hand, and said, "Ya, I do, I was hoping you wouldn't have remembered." At that moment, I realized that the trip was for me. Angelo had thought it through when he made the plans, it was meant to get me away from it all. We said nothing more about it that day, but I was sad and miserable. I knew I had to put my best foot forward, if not for me then for Angelo. We did not need to say anymore about it, we just had to look at each other and we both knew. Angelo and I felt a special kind of bond, the bond you feel with someone after you have gone through a traumatic ordeal. I knew, in my heart that no one understood my pain except for Angelo. Our love for each other became stronger and more intense, not to mention our compassion for each other's feelings.

We saw gorgeous waterfalls and deer crossing the road. "Look mommy, that deer has three children just like you." Joseph said, "Yup, but my deer are cuter than hers." Gaetano sat up and exclaimed, "We're not deer we're humans." Angelo and I laughed. We found exciting caves and teepees but no Indians. The children kept looking for them. We were heading home in a few days and were on the road a lot. Finally, I spotted a sign "Traditional Pow Wow." "Hey follow that sign." I yelled. Angelo turned on to a dirt road and the children asked, "What's happening?" "We found a real Pow Wow." I said. Everyone began to cheer; they were so excited.

There were people wearing traditional Indian outfits, with bright and vivacious colors, women with beautiful shiny black hair and deep eyes, and men wearing beads and feathers. There were booths selling dream catchers in every size imaginable. I bought feathers to put in Lucy's hair. She was so cute with her blond hair full of colorful feathers. We stayed there for most of the day and watched the traditional dances. Everyone was very friendly and allowed us to take pictures of them. We bought five dream catchers and two porcelain dolls dressed in traditional leather Indian outfits. It was a wonderful day and we would be heading home in the morning. It was a bittersweet vacation. We had so much fun bonding yet I was sad.

For the rest of the summer Angelo worked and I took the children to the beach every day. The children were happy playing in the water and building sand castles. Joseph became himself again, and I made every effort for him to feel that everything was back to normal. I hid my feelings well, but I made sure they wore life jackets and they never left my sight. I continued to wait for a big bolt of lighting to come and cause tragedy once again; I continued to wait for judgment day.

- 21 -
Holidays

Joseph had started grade one and Halloween was well on its way. All three kids had specific ideas for their costumes so I got out the sewing machine. I sewed a Dracula outfit for Joseph. I painted his face white and poured stage blood all over his mouth, chin, and his white shirt. Gaetano wanted to be Harry Potter and I had to watch the movie to take notes of his clothing. I sewed a black overcoat and bought him a short black wig. Gaetano was extremely excited when I showed him the round black glasses he was about to wear and the wand he was to hold. Lucy was a witch, but I made sure she was the cutest witch ever. I pictured her as a little Tabatha from "Bewitched." I curled her blond hair and dressed her in a shiny witch's dress. I tried to be happy, but I kept thinking of Luca. If he were here, I probably would have made him a doggy outfit or whatever he wanted, but no matter what my feelings and thoughts were, I still had three children that deserved my time and energy. I dressed up as Tammy Faye and Angelo was a pirate and we entered the world of make believe.

Christmas was one of the toughest holidays for me. The children had helped me decorate the Christmas tree weeks earlier. Every day they asked, "When is Santa coming?" Joseph's list grew longer by the day, and I spent days preparing a shopping list for our fish dinner. Christmas morning finally arrived and the children ran down the stairs to see if all their wishes had come true. I was happy knowing that the rest of the day would be spent cooking our favorite fish dishes and I could eat and eat and eat. I did not want to be happy. One of my sons was not there to open a gift and I did not feel like celebrating. I made all of our traditional fish recipes, starting with stuffed calamari cooked in red sauce. I sautéed butter, white wine, and garlic with clams and waited for the right moment to throw in cooked linguini. The aroma filled the room as I battered and deep-fried lots of large shrimp. I finished it all off with a Greek salad. The aroma of basil and garlic lingered the entire day. As usual, I made enough fish to feed an army, but an army of five not six. Angelo laughed at me and said, "You're so cute. Once again you cooked too much, but I'm not complaining."

Everyone grabbed for their favorite dish. Angelo started with the stuffed squid "Oh my God. I love this." Joseph fought his way to the linguini and gorged as though there was no tomorrow. Gaetano carefully picked the batter off the shrimp and I laughed as he got excited when he found the shrimp. Lucy used her hands to pick at the linguini and let the sauce pour down her top. As for me, well I just wanted to make my family happy and I knew this was the way to their hearts. Though something bothered me the entire day and I knew that eventually I would have to talk to Angelo about it. I waited until everyone had settled into the evening, and I told him that I needed to talk. I lowered the volume on the television, and he knew I was serious. "Ang, the kids got so many gifts, but do you think we should do something in the memory of the baby?" He sat up and said, "Ant, if its important to you, go ahead and do what you gotta do, but we need to let this go." I began to cry out of frustration and replied, "How, how do we let it go? Every Downs child I see, I think, what if. Were we considering him or us? I can't let go, I can't forget, and I can't forgive." I continued to cry and the tears felt as heavy as they did the day it all started. Angelo gave me a hug, "Think of something that will honor him, and do it."

After the holidays I focused on my task immediately, but nothing caught my attention. I wondered around the house looking for ideas and my frustration increased. "Come on Ant, think. What gift could I possibly give Luca that would be special? Think." I sat at the kitchen table and thought, "It can't be an object. How about a donation to the church?" but I wanted the gift to reflect Luca, not the church. "How about a donation to the Downs syndrome society?" I went through the yellow pages and searched for a program that researched Down's. I could not find a page that offered even a hint of where to search, so I called the city of Toronto office and asked, "Do you have the phone number of the Down's Syndrome society?" "Is this for information?" The woman asked. "No, I would like to give a donation." As I said the word donation, I felt happy. I knew I was giving money to a good cause and I felt very proud to have this conversation. "Yes, I do have a number." She said. I happily wrote it down and could not wait another minute to make the call. I felt as though I was giving Luca a wonderful Christmas gift. A soft voice replied. I pictured her as an older woman slim, and petite, with black short hair.

"I would like to give a donation of $100." then I added, "I will be making this donation every Christmas." The woman's voice rose and I could feel her smile. When she said, "We could use all the donations we can get. We are truly grateful for people like you." She then asked, "Do you have a preference as to where you want the money to go?" "What are the options?" I replied, "Well, we can put it towards their education or supplies needed." I stopped her and asked, "Is there any kind of research being done as to why this happens?" "There is a lab trying to come up with answers." She answered. "That's were I want the money to go." She then caught me off guard and asked, "Do you have a Down syndrome child?" I was flustered and searched for a very quick answer, but I did not know what to say. I did not want to be judged and I had learned my lesson about flapping my mouth, so I politely said, "No, I just have a personal reason for my donation." I became quiet and did not offer any more information.

I was happy and, looking up at the ceiling, I quietly mouthed "Merry Christmas Luca", so the children would not hear me. I wanted to tell someone of my good deed and I thought, "Ang should know." I dialed his number at work and said, "Ang, I just donated $100.00 to the Down's Society. Wasn't that a great idea?" I could feel my smile reach from ear to ear. "That's great baby, but I have to get back to work." His voice did not sound happy, and I knew he could not share in my excitement. "What's wrong?" He answered abruptly, "Ant, I'm working, I've got to go." Tears began to form in my eyes and once again I looked up to the ceiling and quietly said, "Daddy wishes you a Merry Christmas too baby."

I began to notice that Angelo just wanted to forget about everything. He no longer wanted to talk about Luca and I was trying to find a way to hold on. Our thoughts went in different directions, but every once in a while we would come together and Angelo would find a way to express his sadness.

The holidays came and went a few times and I always found a moment to think of Luca and include him in my heart, while the children were having fun. I felt empty inside when I thought he was no longer a topic of conversation for anyone but me. I still tried to bring Luca up in conversation with new acquaintances, always searching to get their approval. I listened to songs on the radio and hung on to every word hoping that someone out there knew how I felt. I continued to feel ashamed, but I no longer spent my time searching for answers. I merely existed for the sake of my husband and my children. I ate constantly hoping to fill the emptiness in my heart. Sadly, the only thing my meals filled was my stomach and my behind as I watched a lot of television.

On the "Montel Show" one day, Silvia Brown consoled a woman who had lost a pregnancy. I raised the volume "Not all babies are meant to be born." She said. I thought about her words. Could this be true? Did God need more Angels? Did God think I was strong enough to send him back or did God think I was weak and knew I did not know how to raise him? Would God give me something I could not handle? Could that be the answer? I began to question myself again, and was afraid. I just did not know if God saw me as strong or weak. This raised more issues and I did not know what to think or what to do about it, for that matter.

I wanted to spend the day in bed. I tried to think of something exciting for the day, but I knew it was just another day. The children came in and jumped on the bed, "We're hungry." I rubbed my eyes and said, "Ya, ya, I know all of you want food." I was annoyed that the children needed my attention. I felt annoyed that I had to deal with another day. I got up and washed my face, put my hair in a big ponytail, and dressed in the same clothes I wore the day before. I looked down at my top and noticed an oil stain, "Ah, to hell with it, who cares." I did not think about my appearance anymore, after all, I was fat and nothing looked good on me anyway, so why bother trying. Angelo always said he loved me no matter how much I weighed and that encouraged me to eat more. My sadness carried me through the day. It was easier to feel miserable than to put energy into being happy, happy, happy.

Gaetano chased Lucy and they tried to outrun each other. They were having such a great time but I started yelling,

"Find something quiet to do. The noise is getting on my nerves." The children stopped running and I could hear them whisper to each other, "We're getting on moms nerves." "I didn't say you were getting on my nerves, I said the noise was." I yelled. The children did not give a thought to my words and walked away. I felt terrible. They were just having fun, but I could not handle it. I had forgotten how to appreciate the littlest things in life, including my children's laughter or my husband's caresses. Before I knew it, thank God, it was time for bed.

- 22 -

Home Alone

September 2006 the children dressed for their first day at school. Joseph was starting grade three now and he was very excited. He wore a new pair of jeans and fussed over the laces on his new runners. I walked into Gaetano's bedroom hoping he was putting on the clothes I had laid out for him, but I stopped when I heard him say, "Lucy, just follow me, I'll show you to your classroom." "But Gaetano, will my teacher be mean to me?" She asked. "No, she will be nice, if you listen to the rules." He paused for a moment and added, "Lucy, trust me, I'm in senior kindergarten now, I know what I'm talking about." I was so proud of Gaetano and I knew Lucy would be well taken care of at school by her big brother. Lucy wore a lime green skirt with a matching top. "Lucy you look great. Gaetano I'm proud of you for letting Lucy know school is fun, and by the way, you look handsome." The children grabbed their backpacks and I grabbed the camera. I was so excited for them and I thought, "This will be the first time in eight years that I will have some time to myself." The children posed and I clicked away until Joseph said, "Enough already." I drove them to school and kissed them good-bye. As they walked up the path to the school doors, I followed them with a video camera. Joseph ran as fast as he could and I could hear him yell, "You're so embarrassing." I yelled back, "No. I'm your mamma." I managed to follow the two little ones and waived until I could no longer see them.

I drove home thinking, "Now I have time to talk on the phone with no interruptions. Who should I call first?" I felt old at 41 and I did not have many close friends in the suburbs. I still had a lot of friends in the city to call, but everyone had had their share of my tears and I did not want to cry on their shoulders anymore. "Maybe I'll get some laundry done. No, I know, I'll watch a movie right in the middle of the day." I giggled at the idea but dismissed it pretty quickly; I had better things to do. "Maybe I'll start my journal, write a book about Luca." I drove up to the house and looked around, not a person in sight and it felt like a ghost town. My neighbors minded their own business for the most part, so there really were no personal relationships there either, and I tried my hardest to come up with something exciting to do. I began to fantasize about my journal and I began to think of all the sadness that came with my story. I imagined myself sitting on stage with Oprah. Her praising my wonderful story and telling the audience to read my book.

"This book is empowering." Oprah said and everyone applauded. My fantasy motivated me to get started.

I found myself facing a quiet lonely house. No sound came from the television nor were any toys being thrown around. None of the children were there to ask for my time, and, most of all, no one needed my attention. I found myself picking up the phone book and going from A to Z, trying to find someone to call. I leafed through the pages, waiting for a name to pop up, but it did not happen. I lay on the sofa and tried to breath deeply, enjoy the calmness, but my mind was racing. I kept thinking that all of my attention would have been on Luca now if he were here. I wondered if he was in heaven playing or was he looking down at me saying, you deserve to be alone. I felt nauseous and I needed to keep my mind busy or I would drive myself crazy. What do I do with myself now? I started dinner at 11:00 AM, then washed the floor. I yelled out loud, "I just washed the floor, no one walk around until it's dried." Then I giggled, knowing I was talking to the walls. The phone did not ring for the entire day and I was relieved when 3:00 PM arrived and it was time to pick up my children.

I did not look forward to the days of quiet ahead and I especially dreaded the loneliness. I did not feel like having an espresso that morning, I just wanted a regular coffee. The drive to school would waste a good half hour before I headed home. I opened the front door and called out, "Honey I'm home." I smirked as I looked into the hallway. The children had left a pile of shoes next to the shoebox and I stared at the dry mud left behind from Angelo's construction boots. I closed the front door behind me and bent down to pick up the shoes, but I felt a rage come over me. The shoe in my hand felt heavy and I used every bit of strength to squeeze it. I yelled out loud, "Please Jesus save me." I fell to my knees and cried until my head began to throb, and I knew I had drained all of my anger out. I wiped my face with my sleeve and said, "God why can't I get over this? It's been years now and I still can't forgive myself." I started to think of my neighbor across the street and decided that I needed some company. I found it odd to be thinking of Dina, but at the same time, I really wanted to call. I knew there would be a flow of conversations between us, because we did not really know each other very well. I felt nervous dialing her number, I did not want a rejection of my visit, but more than anything I did not want to be alone.

"Hey Dina." Her voice rose and I could sense she had a smile on her face as she replied, "Hey Ant, how are you?" "I'm good, listen I just bought myself a coffee and I was wondering if you felt like having company?" Dina was a quiet woman and when we had spoken briefly in the past, she always seemed very quiet and reserved. She did not hesitate and replied, "Ya, give me half an hour and come over."

Dina stood at the door with a big smile and welcomed me in. She was a tall slender woman, with light brown hair she wore in a ponytail and hung over her shoulder. "Dina your house looks like it came out of a magazine." I exclaimed. We sat at the kitchen table and I was careful not to put my fingerprints on the glass. "Dina are you still

working part time?" "No not right now, I need a break."
She replied. We gossiped for a while about people in our
neighborhood and it did not take long before I began to
speak of Luca. My mind told me to be quiet and keep
my business to myself. I knew Angelo would not have
approved but my heart was exploding. No one wanted to
hear about my son anymore, but I was not done. I needed
to talk about him, I needed to remember every detail to
keep my son alive. I could feel my headache return as I
released the words and revealed every detail of my dirty
secret. I cried and choked on my words as I tried to bring
her to the moment of our family feud, and I cried about
my broken heart that just lies in my body and pumps old
dark blood.

Dina gave me her undivided attention and just listened
until I had tired myself out. It struck me that she did
not say very much, and I looked at her wondering if she
thought I was a nut case. I wiped away my tears and said,
"I apologize for my performance." She gave me a warm
smile and asked, "Can I give you an Angel reading?"
"What's an Angel reading?" I asked. "Do you believe in
Angels?" "Yes." I became excited and said, "Is it like tarot
cards?" Dina laughed and replied, "Something like that,
but it's a reading from the Angels." She brought out a
box, slightly larger than a deck of cards, and placed the
cards on the table as she sat next to me. I could not stop
staring at the box and the beautiful Angel on its cover.
The colors were vibrant and the Angel's face reminded
me of a porcelain doll. She pulled the cards out of the
deck and said, "Okay, shuffle them well." "Okay why not,
what could a deck of cards possibly tell me?" I thought

and shuffled each card thinking that if I shuffled well the results would be amazing. As I shuffled Dina told me to ask the Angels to remove anyone else's oracles from the cards. "What's an oracle?" I asked. "You're just asking the Angels to come around you and not the last person who touched the cards." She continued, "Repeat after me," I listened carefully as she began, "Dear Angels please guide my reading so that it is in the light and is accurate. Please help me to understand my reading so that it is specific and benefits everyone involved." I listened carefully to every word as I repeated it. "Fan the cards open, leaning them on your chest, on your heart and ask the Angels a question." "Do I ask my question out loud?" "Whatever you're comfortable with." I chose to share my question with Dina and asked, "Angels, has God forgiven me for my sin?" Dina then instructed me to choose three cards and place them face up on the table. She began my reading with the guidance of a book.

The first card was entitled, "All is forgiven." I felt a shiver run down my spine and as Dina read the card I interpreted it to say that God loves me and that I have been forgiven. She said that I need to forgive myself and move on. Dina stopped for a moment as she searched for the page that explained the second card. The second card advised me to stop explaining myself to everyone and to stop trying to get everyone's approval. Dina asked me, "Are you ready for the last one?" I could not believe the power the cards had over me and I wanted more. I said, "Yes please." The card revealed that I had a fantastic idea that I needed to put into motion. Dina stopped reading and asked, "Do you know what the Angels are referring to?" I started to laugh and cry at the same time and said, "I do, I want to write a book about my story!" Dina smiled and said, "I think the Angels are steering you this way." I could not believe what I was hearing and asked, "Is someone out there really listening to me?"

It was getting late and I had to pick up the children from school. "You know Dina, I have no idea what made me call you. But I'm happy I did." "Ant I give myself an Angel reading every morning, and this morning the cards told me I needed to help someone today. I didn't understand who I was supposed to teach until you called." She said.

I was drained, my face felt red and hot, my eyes were puffy from all the tears, but I felt good and very sleepy. I walked home thinking, "What the hell just happened?" I could not get these cards out of my mind.

My mind dwelled on the day's events and I knew I had to get a deck of cards for myself. I kept hearing Dina tell me about the laws of attraction, and how my negative thoughts attract the universe. I thought to myself, "Think positively, I must change my ways." I thought, "If I believe the baby is in heaven with God and my dad, then will it be true? Does this mean the entire time I kept thinking he was lonely and cold in the ground that I willed this?" I needed more knowledge about the cards and I needed more answers to my questions.

That evening, after dinner, the children went to the playroom, and Angelo watched television. "Angelo I went over to Dina's today." I said. Angelo looked up, "What did you guys talk about?" He lowered the volume and gave me his undivided attention. "Well, I just needed to talk and I told her about the baby." Angelo sat up, "Ant, I thought we weren't going to talk about that anymore." I began to explain to him about the Angel cards but I could tell he was not a believer. "You seem very excited about these cards." "Angelo, they made me feel like God and the Angel's were listening to me." "That's great hun." He raised the volume and focused his attention to the television. I wanted him to be excited too, but that just did not happen.

- 23 -

In Search of Angels

The morning was a mad rush to get the children dressed. Lucy was the fastest. Gaetano had his pants up and one sock on, while he played with his game-boy. I kept saying, "Gaetano, please, you need to get to school. Put the game-boy down and get dressed." Joseph walked around holding his toothbrush. I was frustrated. My mind was on getting them to school so I could scurry downtown and find the store that sold the Angel cards. I waved good-bye to the children and the excitement took over my body. I felt as though I had finally found some answers, or at the very least some higher power that would actually answer me. I drove up and down the street with the country station blaring. For the first time in a long time, I sang from the top of my lungs. I could not find the store and, finally I stopped and asked for directions. They looked at me and pointed over to a little store five feet away. I started to

giggle and said, "Thanks, I guess I was looking too hard."
I could not believe that in my anticipation it was in front
of my eyes and yet so far. There was so much to see in
the store that I became slightly overwhelmed. I started
to look at every corner and I felt calm and safe. I knew I
needed to be here and I took my time.

Dream catchers were hanging from the ceiling and walls.
The shelves were full of shiny rocks and stones of all
colors. I had no idea what they meant, but I was overjoyed
and wanted to understand. I walked over to a corner in
the back of the store with many statues of Angels and
fairies and wizards. My eyes lit up at the beauty, I did not
want to leave. The lighting was dim with candles burning
everywhere and the walls were a quiet surreal color. At
the back of the room a large blue cloth printed with stars
and moons hung from the ceiling in a circle, creating a
round room. A corner of the curtain was pulled back and
I could see a little table in the center. I knew it was for
psychic readings. I was excited and thought, "I wonder if
the psychic is in today for a reading." I was familiar with
readings and had done them often in the past.

Growing up I was always interested in psychic readings
and believed psychics had special powers to know the past,
present, and future. My friends always said I was gullible,
but how did psychics know so much about me when I
never uttered a word? I always knew there were answers
in the universe and I spent my entire life trying to figure
things out. My thoughts about psychics were interrupted
when a woman came over and asked me if she could help.
I had not even turned to face her yet I felt a sense of calm.

I just wanted to take her by the hand, drag her to the front of the store, and say, "Let's start from the beginning of the store. You need to teach me everything you know." I wanted so desperately to learn everything. I was starved for her knowledge; maybe she had answers to everything, to anything, to something.

She was a young woman with long shiny black hair. Her eyes were a piercing green and she wore dark clothing. She wore a necklace with a stone that she rubbed back and forth as she gave me her full attention. "Do you have Angel cards?" I asked. "Yes." She answered as she headed towards the counter. There they were on a shelf. There were numerous boxes of all colors and I did not know which one exactly I was looking for. "I'm not sure which one to buy." I said. She put a few decks on the table. I looked at a yellowish gold box with a soothing Angel on its cover and it felt good to stare at her. The next box was pale blue and had dolphins on it, but I had no idea why anyone would ask dolphins for answers to anything. The box next to it was dark blue and had a wizard on it and I felt drawn to it, but not in a good way. I was uneasy but I kept staring at it.

She caught my eye staring at the box and asked me, "Do you feel an easy calm when you look at the wizard box?" "Actually I feel uneasy and yet curious." The young woman put her hand over the deck and said, "This isn't for you then, take a look at the others and tell me which one you are drawn to with comfort and ease." I looked once again and stared at the remaining three decks and pointed to the gold box with beautiful Angels. She picked up the deck and said, "This is the one that was calling out to you. You need to start off with these."

I began to look around again. I honestly did not want to leave. I knew there was something about this place that I needed and I needed to stay. I went over to the shelf with the colored stones and I stared at all the beautiful colors. "I wonder if Dina could teach me about these stones." I decided to buy Dina a stone to thank her for helping me find that little bit of hope I had lost and was so desperate to find again. I picked up a purple stone and a purple case to put it in. The saleswoman cleaned the stone with oil and told me, "The person who owns it should be the only one to touch the stone from this point." "What can I tell her it is?' I asked. She smiled, "If she understands astrology she will know, but if you feel a need to tell her something, just say it's a Lapis Lazuli stone, the third eye." She added, "The Internet can explain that this stone is for love, fidelity, and peace. She should lie down in a quiet room and meditate with this stone on her forehead and it will give her new insights." My business at the store was complete. I left with great hesitation but I was excited to go home and try out my new Angel cards. As I walked to the van I wanted to tell strangers, "Look, look at what I bought. You should get it too. It really works. It will give you answers." But, of course, I walked quietly to my van and drove home.

I ran into the house, threw my purse and coat on the floor, and ran to the dining room table. I did not pay attention to the shoes and coats lying around in the hallway or even the breakfast dishes still sitting on the dining room table.

I ripped open the plastic and pulled the deck out of the box. I rubbed every card so that my scent would be on them and shuffled them as best as I could. I raised the deck up to my heart, fanned the cards and said, "Dear Angels, please clear my mind to get an accurate reading and help me to understand what you want me to know." I chose three cards and placed them on the table, one by one, from left to right.

The first card said that I was loved and needed to love myself. It said I needed to stop punishing myself for the past and move on. Tears swelled in my eyes, because I wanted to believe that the cards were referring to Luca. I needed more and searched through the book to find the significance of the second card. The second card said that the future was bright for me and I needed to bring out the child in me and go play. Take a walk, go down a slide, just enjoy and put aside all my worries. The third card was the "Brilliant Idea" card. I stared at it and said out loud, "Angels, are you referring to my book?" I began to read and the book told me that I had a brilliant idea that I needed to manifest and I, as well as others would prosper from it. It went on to tell me that an abundance of gold and fortune, in many different forms, would come my way, but I needed to begin my task. I thought, "in many different forms." Will it be money or peace of mind?'

I began to feel a sense of calm. I needed something to believe in, and the cards gave me the attention I was looking for. I felt truly blessed when I read the cards and my heart pounded fast when I held them. I was excited. I went on with my daily routine, but I now had something exciting to look forward to. I kept telling myself, "You heard the Angels. Write a book." As I washed dishes, I thought of stories I could write and doing the laundry, I thought of how I was raised. I began to laugh when I thought of the fun times I had with my sisters. I tried to fight the demons that entered my mind and the fear that followed. I felt shaky and nervous "What if people rally outside my door and try to ban this book? What if I put my family in jeopardy over this? The bottom line is, I aborted my son." I tried to reason with myself, "What if someone else is going through the same thing?" Maybe some good could come out of all this." I did not want to add any more pain to my family and I certainly did not want to start any more family wars.

That evening I went to bed and I could not get the book out of my mind. A tennis match went on in my mind. I went back and forth with the pros and cons and I needed validation for my idea. I just wanted to tell someone my story and reach out to someone who was in pain too. Then I thought, "Even if I can't help anyone, maybe I can tell the world that God forgives, or at least I hope he does." Eventually my fears overpowered my excitement and I decided to write my story in a personal journal that my children could read one day. I wrote every word without much thought. I just wrote the first thing that made me laugh or cry. I wrote every feeling that made me so mad that I wanted to break something. I even wrote terrible thoughts that I was ashamed to share with anyone. But all the words were mine and I needed to write.

- 24 -
A Flower Girl

My nephew Simon announced he was getting married. Simon, along with his fiancé, invited Lucy to be the flower girl. We were all very excited. Lucy was especially honored to have such a big part in the wedding and secretly, so was I. I kept telling Lucy, "Now you will be the most beautiful princess at the party." "Will everyone be looking at me?" She asked. "Of course." I was happy for my daughter and she felt very important. I knew that from now until the day of the wedding there would be many projects, like dress fittings to complete and parties to attend.

The day came for the bride's wedding shower and Stella was very excited. She had put a lot of thought and planning into this function. "Stella do you want me to take the pictures at the shower?" I knew this would be one less worry on her mind. "Oh, that would be great!"

She replied. I took a lot of pride in my daughter's role and dressed her in a beautiful chiffon skirt with a white top and a little chiffon jacket. She wore her beautiful blond hair down with her bangs pinned back. Lucy was so excited and asked, "Mommy, can I wear lipstick?" I laughed with delight. Lucy was such a girly girl and I was pleased. I graciously said, Okay, you're four, so you can wear a shiny lip gloss." We found a shiny strawberry flavored gloss in my vanity table, and I gently put some on her tiny red lips. Lucy swooshed her lips together and off we went.

There had not been many family functions since my personal tragedy and it was a day that all my sisters and cousins would be together in one room. I kept thinking, "Everyone is going to be looking at me and thinking, she was pregnant with a Down's child." I wanted to show everyone, that I still had a perfect family and it was my chance to show off one of my children and show everyone how perfect she was. I was proud and I knew that if I kept busy with the pictures no one would really have a chance to tell me how great I looked, knowing they were thinking "poor thing, look how heavy she's become due to her heartache." I had become very self-conscious, but more sadly, I had become self-absorbed.

I sat at the table with my sisters and we spoke of nothing important enjoying each other's company. I noticed a Down's girl at another table. She was wearing a pretty white dress and her hair was nicely combed. She was very overweight and I knew she was probably in her mid 30's. She did not leave her chair the entire afternoon nor did her mother leave her side. I watched everyone at her table bring her food, serve her drinks, and cater to her every need, yet not one person sat and had a conversation with her. She just ate and kept her eyes down for the most part. She had sad eyes and seemed quite tired. I could not help but feel sad for her. "Why shouldn't I have saved my son from this? I am his mother, was it not my job to offer him the best I could give?"

I thought about the news and remembered the story of a mother who drowned her five children. She was convinced her children were not safe and she needed to get them to heaven to save them. I once thought that she did not deserve to have children. Although her decision was to the extreme, I now understood the strength of a mother's love, and the desperation to protect her babies. We all try to give our children a good life and protect them from evil. I did what I had to do to protect my son. My inner demons came forward and I thought, "Was I just trying to save us? Am I relieved for Luca or for us?" I felt ashamed of my thoughts and tears formed in my eyes. I started thinking of my father when he was very ill. My father died on Christmas morning in 1996. He was 77 years old and we all took his loss very hard even though he was sick for five years and close to being bed ridden. My mother suffered a couple of strokes trying to take care of him, yet he was worth it. When my father died I could not help feeling sad for myself, but I was so happy for him, he no longer had to suffer. All I could think of was how his mind was alert right to the moment of his death but his body had failed him years before. The big, tall strong man I used to look up to became a tiny frail man. I was happy he was free to walk and run once again. I wanted this happiness for Luca, even if it meant letting him go.

My father always told us, never break the law and always follow the laws of the church. I felt sad thinking that my father was looking down at me with shame. These thoughts went through my mind while I stared at the girl quietly sitting in her chair. Watching her sadness confirmed what I had not wanted for my son. I never wanted to see that sadness in his eyes because of my greed to keep him.

I tried to stare unnoticed but my sister Maria caught my eye. "Anne, I'm very proud of you and your daughter looks gorgeous." Maria followed my stare and said, "Stop worrying about others." I gave Maria a gentle smile with glossy eyes and I knew she could feel my sadness. I tried to hold my breath so the crying sounds would not escape my mouth. I thought that if I did not try to talk the tears would stop. "You need to get over this and move on." Maria said. I just did not know what her words meant. I needed to punish myself every day or God would be mad at me "Mar, I want to write a book on everything that happened." I said and waited for her reaction. Without a moment's hesitation she said, "You should, and I hope you go for it." I was very relieved and thought that maybe I could really do it, maybe it was possible. I began to think that either God had bigger plans for me or I was an idiot trying to air my dirty laundry to the world.

The buffet table was about to close and I wanted to stuff my face with my third plate of pasta. I could see my mother watching me, from the corner of my eye. She shook her head and I knew she was not too happy with my eating habits. "I'm just not going to look at her." I thought and remembered how, when I was a child, on Sunday mornings, my mother went to the 9:00 AM mass. She would come home and start cooking tomato sauce while we got ready for the 11:00 AM mass with my father. He always wore his black fedora and took it off when he entered the church. After church we hurried home, knowing that the pasta was ready. The aroma of fresh basil and plum tomatoes filled our nostrils. The table was set with red wine, and a bowl full of spaghetti waited for us. It was heaven to eat. This was our Sunday, our day of rest.

- 25 -
Good Night my Angels

Weeks went by and I constantly gave myself Angel readings. I wanted the Angels to tell me what to do, how to think and how I was supposed to feel. The cards always referred to the same intent. I was told that God loves and forgives me. I was encouraged to bring out the happy side of myself and to work on my "Brilliant Idea." I knew the Angels were referring to my need to write, yet two years had passed and I had not yet written a word.

I called Dina a few times for reassurance, and as usual, she was non-judgmental and only gave me hope. I always felt better when I spoke to her and my belief in the Angels increased. I tried to include Angelo in the readings, but he was very skeptical and always took the information with a grain of salt. I decided to introduce the Angels to the children. They knew of the Angels but I wanted them to really believe in them, so I came up with a game. I told the children, "let's play a new game." I got their attention and said, "Let's thank God and the Angels for one thing for the day." Lucy sat up and said, "I thank God and the Angels for my barbies." Gaetano was thankful for his game boy and Joseph was grateful for no homework. I laughed and said, "Good job guys." I never corrected them because these were their thoughts and they needed to be accepted. The children played the game every day and took a liking to it.

One evening when I was about to tell a bedtime story I decided to introduce the Angels to the story of Jacomino and Pasqualino. I told the children how Jacomino would close his eyes and the Angels would put their arms around him and hold him. Jacomino asked the Angels to do the same for his brother Pasqualino and his sister Laduika. The children were very excited and added their thoughts to the story. We closed our eyes and asked the Angels to do the same for us. "Mommy, I could see the Angels." The children said. "What color are they wearing?" I asked, "They're wearing bright pink and purple and they have red lipstick on." Lucy answered. Joseph did not allow her to finish, and said, "No, they're wearing Toronto Maple Leaf shirts." I entertained his idea and said, "That's cool." Then of course, it was Gaetano's turn. He was very excited. His eyes lit up and he said, "Mommy did you know the Angels fly around at night to save the souls of all the children?" "Gaetano, is that true?" I asked. He came closer to me, putting his little face close to mine and said, "Ya, and I help them. I climb out of my window at night and I fly around and help the Angels." I could not believe his story but I said, "Wow that's amazing." Gaetano added, "Why do you think I'm so tired in the morning for school?' I laughed, "Well, now I know." He was pleased and content with his idea.

Lucy and Gaetano were still small enough to be happy over the simplest pleasures, including a bedtime story. Joseph was very different and would take every word to heart. He would always turn everything into a negative. I knew he was following my path and I had to change his ways. I prayed that my children would never take on my negative ideas and I needed to make sure that they did not repeat me. I decided to "walk the walk and talk the talk." I knew Joseph thought my stories were silly, but I did not care, I just kept reminding him that the Angels were around. I believed in God and the Angels and of course the Saints but I had gone against all of my beliefs with my decisions. I certainly had no right to ask for forgiveness.

My soul was in a hopeless situation but my children's souls were still small and tender, and I knew I could mold them to believe in the greater good. More importantly, I needed them to believe that they could not look for external validation but had to find it within themselves. My children were now my goal and my focus.

- 26 -
A Dream

I dreamt that I was sitting in Dina's garage. I sat on a small pink sofa and waited for her to come and join me. Her husband walked into the garage and asked me what I was doing there. I sat up and told him that I was waiting for Dina, she had gone into the kitchen to get me a surprise. I felt a sense of happiness and there was nothing negative in the dream. I woke up in the morning and wondered what it all meant.

The snow was falling down quite heavily and Angelo went out to shovel. I stood outside on the veranda in my slippers. The cold wind brushed by me and light snowflakes landed on my shoulders. I had such a desire to stand there and just watch him as he used all his strength to pull the cord and get the motor on the snow blower started. I always felt an emotional bond to Angelo when I watched him do his tasks and, of course, he always had a cigarette hanging from the side of his lips. A warm espresso kept my hands warm. I just watched Angelo and felt truly blessed. I closed my eyes and pictured the Angels holding hands in a circle around me. I pictured them floating around and around me, and I felt light and carefree. I opened my eyes and looked up at the sky. "I wonder if Luca can feel snow in heaven, or is he just cold in his grave." I tried to focus my thoughts elsewhere, when I noticed Dina across the street.

I quickly ran into the house, slipped my boots on and grabbed my jacket. I was excited to tell her about my dream and ask her what she thought it meant. "We all felt happy and you had a present for me." I told her. Dina just kept saying, "Oh my God." Her eyes opened wide and she said, "Go look in my garage." As I started walking towards her garage, a small part of me thought, "Could there be a pink sofa in there?" I looked in and there it was, a love seat and it was pink. I started laughing and said, "Oh my God, Dina, do you think the dream was referring to the readings? Do you think that was what you went into the kitchen for?" "Ant, I did buy you a gift, but I was waiting for the right time to give it to you, and now is the time." she said, "Come in for a coffee." and we went into the house.

I sat at her kitchen table and she brought the gift all wrapped up with a bow. She handed it to me and I could not wait to tear the paper off. I knew in my heart it would be something spiritual and my anticipation was at an all time high. I could never have imagined what was about to happen. It was a book by Doreen Virtue entitled,

"Daily Guidance from your Angels." The cover was a deep purple and had an Angel with her wings straight out into the air. The Angel was riding a beautiful white unicorn and she had an intense expression on her face. Her face was porcelain and she had flowers around her hair. She wore a pink flowing gown. The cover was gorgeous and I could not stop saying, "Thank you, this is beautiful." I could tell Dina was very pleased with herself. I realized, at that moment, she was on her own personal mission and helping others was her calling.

"I was at the bookstore and the Angels were telling me that I needed to buy this book for you." "Should I open to a page and read?" I asked gratefully and, not waiting for her answer chose a page that felt right. "Stop procrastinating" it read, I should begin my "Brilliant Idea." The Angels told me to start writing from the beginning or the middle or the end, it did not matter where I started as long as I started. They said that if I wrote down some words, the story would manifest itself and would come to life on its own. The Angels also told me not to worry what anyone thought, because they were guiding me and protecting me. I closed the book and Dina said, "You haven't started writing your book, have you?" I nodded and said, "I was afraid someone would try to hurt my family over this book." She smiled, "Well, now you know, don't think about that and just write" she continued, "Those little voices that give you the ideas of what you want to write are all coming from the Angels." Shivers ran down my spine, but I felt safe around her.

Dina gave me a sheet of paper with bright pink, purple, and red hearts around the border. In purple marker she had written: "In the infinity of life where I am, all is perfect, whole and complete." I immediately decided that it was Luca speaking to me. I continued to read, "I am one with the power that created me. I am totally open and receptive to the abundant flow of prosperity that the universe offers. All my needs and desires are met before I even ask. I am divinely guided and protected and I make choices that are beneficial to me. I rejoice in others' successes, knowing there is plenty for all of us. I am constantly increasing my conscious awareness of abundance and this reflects in a constantly increasing income. My good comes from everyone and everywhere. All is well in my world." This poem was powerful for me. I wanted to believe Luca was telling me he was safe with God. I wanted to believe that the universe heard me and that my family was protected. I wanted to believe that I was going to be fine. Many emotions poured over me. Dina waited until I finished reading and said, "Live your life by these words and say them every morning." I tucked the sheet into my beautiful new book and I felt very grateful and very safe. I knew I was now headed into a safer place; maybe this was my saving grace.

- 27 -
A Book is Born

I sat down at the computer, feeling intimidated but I started to type. At first I smiled as I wrote about the children and Angelo. Before I knew it, I had written a few pages and it all made sense. I felt a sense of relief and began to think it may actually happen. I was proud of what I had written and sat at the computer for hours. The more I wrote, the more I thought of, and my fingers clicked away, word after word day after day.

Angelo knew how important this book was to me. He made every effort to start dinner and had the children clean the kitchen table. Many times Angelo asked, "Do you think you could shut down the computer and spend time with me?" I felt guilty for leaving him alone in front of the television but when I was with him, my mind was upstairs in front of the computer. I did not have much time to write when the children were around, because they followed me like lost puppies and I was always distracted. I made a point of writing late at night, when the children were asleep and Angelo had nodded off in front of the television.

It became easy to pour my heart out on paper and I had so much to say. Not only did the pages come to life, but so did the painful feelings. I could feel my heart break all over again and my soul was in turmoil. I cried the entire time I wrote and it felt as though everything was happening all over again. I wanted to bring all the hurt back to life, so I could bring my son back to life again. I did not know if I could continue and so I stopped writing. I had no desire to walk away, because it felt safe here. The yellow curtains with purple stars and moons remained on the window. I stared at it, " How ironic is that." I thought. It felt as though the universe was empowering me to continue my journey and I wanted to believe that Luca was in the room encouraging me to be strong. Year's before I couldn't stand to be in this room now I couldn't imagine leaving.

Stella called, I knew if I told her about my writing I would get an honest opinion. I was not ready to hear it before but I was now. I needed to know whether or not I was doing the right thing. "Stella I'm writing a journal." I said. "Okay, about what?" "Well, about everything that happened to me." "You mean about the baby?" I quietly answered, "Yes." My heart pounded and I felt panicky as I waited for her response. "That's great if it helps you to get over it." After I read her a couple of pages she breathed heavily and said, "That really sounds like you." "I'll help you in any way I can. If you need me to read it over for you, I'll be happy to do that." I felt validated and knew that I should continue writing. "Wow, this abortion has really affected you." She said. I could not continue reading. The words on paper were so real and so alive to me that my voice quivered and I wanted to cry. I wiped my tears, blew my nose and muttered through my laughter. "What did you say?" Stella asked. "I said I can't read any of the pages out loud without crying, and you should see me when I'm writing, I used up a box of Kleenex." We both laughed, "You're going to have the entire family crying when they read your story. I've got to go, but keep me up to date with your book, it's really good."

I spent so much of my time feeling sorry for myself that I had forgotten about Angelo's worries. Another cold winter was settling in. It was getting too cold for cement to be poured and Angelo's job was ending for the season. The men were put on call until spring. He tried to find a part time job to hold us over for the winter, but it was not easy and we became very edgy with each other. I started to work in the evenings as a telemarketer but the pay was not great and it did not really make a big dent in our bills. I began feeling resentful leaving the children. I constantly promised them toys from the dollar stores to compensate for time I was away but Lucy wanted only me. She would run to the door when I was leaving and say, "Mommy hugs and kissy first?" She had tears in her eyes, and I felt guilty all the time. Angelo later told me that she was fine as soon as I walked out the door. Angelo constantly e-mailed his resume and knocked on doors leaving his resume everywhere. I became my old self again, mad and bitter with life, and I walked away from my writing. I stopped reading the Angel cards and my entire focus was on paying our bills. I knew once the season started up again for Angelo, we would be better, but the bills waited for no one, and we both knew we were falling behind.

I went into my bedroom turned off the light, and sat on my bed. I was nervous over our household situation and I wanted some guidance from God. I closed my eyes and pictured the Angels around me holding hands and floating. I told them, "Why are you not helping me? I've put my order out into the universe and all I'm getting are more bills and deeper in debt." I was so angry I did not even ask God and the Angels for help. I yelled at them in my anger. I felt no shame, after all I had kept a positive outlook, I put my order out into the universe and I recieved nothing in return. Somehow it did not seem fair to me that once again I was wronged by God.

I do not remember lying down and falling asleep but I do remember I dreamt about Angelo and me looking for an apartment to live in, but they were all too expensive.

We went to numerous apartments until we found one that fit our budget. I kept telling myself we ran out of money and had to make the best of things. I woke up in a panic. My heart beat wildly in my chest and I was sweating. I knew it would be one of those moody days and I knew I was on a rampage. I got out of bed grabbed the "Daily Guidance" book and said, "You're coming with me." I picked the book up with much anger in my heart but as I walked away the book fell out of my hand and landed open, face down. I stood there for a moment and thought, "Do you want me to read this specific page? Okay then I will." I lifted the book from the floor careful so as not to lose the page and I sat down on the bed.

I looked over to the left side of the book and began to read. The Angels began by telling me that I had steered away from good. I was on the right path, but I had fallen. The Angels advised that I go back to meditating and return to the right path. They also said that they have never left me and still love me. I started to laugh and said out loud, "I can't believe the Angels just told me off." I began to read the right side of the book and I could not believe what I was reading. The Angels told me I had neglected my "Brilliant Idea." I said, "I'm assuming you're talking about writing." They told me that I needed to leave my worries to God and the Angels and just concentrate, they would take care of me. It felt surreal, and I knew the Angels were setting me back on track, but the evil side of me just wanted to burst out and take over. I could not allow this, not any more. Throughout the day I kept thinking, 'Okay, I'm no longer afraid of my debts, because the Angels are helping." The other side of my brain asked "and they are going to help me how?" It was a struggle, but I made a conscious decision to sit at the computer and write, but first I needed to call Dina.

I told her about my dream, and the pages I read. She did not seem surprised. Whenever I spoke to her about my experiences with the Angels, she always discussed the situation with me as a matter of fact. She added, "The Angels don't take breaks, they are always listening." Dina became excited, her voice rose and she said, "Ant, you need to watch Oprah today. Have you heard about the book called The Secret?" "No." I replied. "The guests on Oprah will explain about putting your order out into the universe. Watch it, they're going to explain everything I've been talking about."

- 28 -
The Secret

I made myself an espresso and sat in front of the television with great anticipation. I really needed to find my inner peace and I knew, from watching Oprah for so many years, that she really believed in the Angels and I knew I would benefit from this show. Everyday when 3:00 PM came around, I would burst out and sing the old theme song that used to start Oprah's show. I loved that song and I remember feeling such loss when the song was taken off the air. There was something about it, and to this day it always makes me smile when I sing it. I even incorporated the song into one of my Jacomino and Pasqualino stories, so that the children would learn to sing along as well. Waiting for the commercials to end, I took a deep breath and began to sing 'I see ten thousand stories and glories and dreams, see Angels right here on earth, ooh hoo, our

hearts are open wide, there's a new light shining inside....."
and "Oprah" began.

She had four guests on the show and began to explain "The Secret." I hung on to every word. I repeated what they said and I understood. I needed three key elements to offer the universe: I needed to think it, believe it with all my heart, and I needed to act on it. If I left out any one of these three key players, I would not succeed.

I got it, I got it, I GOT IT!

I started to smile and yelled, "If I believe I can achieve, I got it!" I stood up from the sofa and started doing an "I got it" dance. I wanted to make this my bible and I wanted so desperately to find a better life, after all it could not get any worse. As the show went on, I was already putting my plan into action and I decided that today was the day I would go on a diet to shed my demonic fat. Lose the fat and lose the low self-esteem that goes along with it. I also decided my book would be written. I did not care anymore who was going to read it, because I was going to finish the book for me. If anyone had the opportunity to benefit from it, well, so be it, but I realized that the one person I wanted to save was me. I felt happy and I knew it was going to work. Just as fast as the positive came through my heart so did the negative. My brain tried desperately to push the words out of my mouth, "This is all crap." I fought hard not to utter the words that I knew and cradled so well. I told the Angels they could take my old and negative thoughts and file them under G. I also asked for guidance to help me think, believe and, for once in my life achieve. I started asking the Angels for more guidance and to help me fulfill my new destiny.

The cards along with the Daily Guidance book constantly steered me towards feeling better about myself and gave me specific points to think about. Sometimes they would tell me I was on my way to a better life for me and for those around me. "Luca is not in a cold grave, and he is in heaven happy." I thought and convinced myself that God and my father are surrounding him, and all is well. I lay down and tried to remember all the good that God had done for me and I recalled a time when I was a young child.

I slept in the lower half of the bunk bed and I would always cover my eyes when I was afraid of the dark. I knew my sister Tracey was just above me but I was still afraid and I would close my eyes and say the "Our Father". Then, as soon as I heard a noise, I would quickly open my eyes, afraid that a stranger had come into our room. Of course no one was ever there, and eventually I would fall asleep holding a rosary.

One night, the usual routine began when the lights were shut off. I closed my eyes and said my prayer, then came a sound and I quickly opened my eyes. A strong feeling came over me and I looked above my head onto the wall, where I saw a pair of hands. They looked like a picture on the wall. The right hand was under the left supporting it. Long bell sleeves covered the wrists and everything was purple. Although I quickly covered my eyes with my hands I was not afraid. I knew it was not evil, I knew they were God's hands, and I knew I was safe. I kept thinking,

"Could it be. Did I really see God's hands?" A part of me said this is not normal and I convinced myself to be afraid. I decided to take another peek and looked above my head. He was gone and all that remained was the white wall. I told my mother the next morning and she encouraged me to believe in what I had seen. She also encouraged me to be thankful for witnessing a miracle that people wait all their lives to see. My mother was very religious and I knew that she believed me. For days after that, I heard her on the phone telling my aunts about it.

I truly believe in what I saw that night and I have always held it in my memory. I can still picture the room with the old dark wood dresser and the white walls that were bumpy to the touch. There was a tiny closet with a door for Tracey and me. And an old dresser made out of dark wood, with full sized mirrors on each door. The left mirror had a crack running down it like a snake and there was a picture of Mother Mary covering the hole. I never knew how that mirror broke and I never thought to ask because it had been there forever. I can still feel the desire to re-create that night and at times I close my eyes and picture it all over again. I feel a sense of peace when I see those soft gentle hands. To this day, when I receive the host, I always place my right hand under my left in anticipation. It reminds me of my special little miracle and reminds God that I am still grateful for this experience. I wondered if Luca had the privilege to see God's hands every day. I began to find my faith again, but I was not sure how much I had forgotten.

Dina and I planned to get the children off to school and go to Chapters. I felt especially down that day, worrying about my finances. On the drive there we spoke about Oprah and "The Secret". Our thoughts went everywhere and were intense. Dina treated me to a cappuccino and as we sat she asked, "Did you know that money is a positive force?" She continued, "When I pass money over to someone, I secretly bless the money over to them." I listened as she went on, "There is an abundance of wealth for everyone. We should be happy for those who prosper." I took her words in but I shared with her, "I'm nowhere near blessing anyone who is taking my money." She laughed and we headed for the Angel Isle.

We picked up a few books and read a couple of pages here and there, trying to feel inspired. We read from Doreen Virtue's books, more than others. I did not feel very spiritual that day and decided to catch a movie. I closed the book I was looking at and put it back on the shelf, "D, do you want to catch a movie?" "You mean now?" I started to smile and answered, "Ya, now, let's go see a movie." Dina started to laugh and put her book back on the shelf. As we walked toward the front of the store, Dina grabbed my arm and said, "I've got a better idea, I'm going to buy "The Secret" and we can watch it back at my house." She had a big smile on her face and I could tell she was very pleased with her idea. I laughed at her expression and agreed. "Let's see if they have it, I came last week and they were sold out. If it's sold out then it's not our time to watch it" she said. Dina went over to the counter and we looked at the DVDs sitting on a shelf. Dina grabbed my arm and jumped up and down with excitement.

On the drive back we were full of excitement and anticipation. I kept thinking and praying to God and the Angels to reach out to me and give me more hope. I asked the Angels if they could somehow reach out to me, specifically, so that I could really understand The Secret. We got ourselves comfortable on Dina's sofa and I propped myself up with a couple of pillows so that I would not miss a word. I felt a sense of empowerment right from the start of the show. I hung on to every word and searched for comparisons to my own in every story. Every once in a while, Dina paused the show, so we could discuss it and interpret it with our own thoughts. Dina was well ahead of me in understanding the power of the universe and she enlightened me. My mind wandered every so often, and I knew that I needed to watch the show again another day.

I started to think of how I could I get the most out of the show to change my thoughts and to really transform, and then it happened. An author named Jack Canfield spoke about the book he had written "Chicken Soup for the Soul." He did not know how to write a book or even where to get it published, but he just knew he had to write it. He spoke of how good he felt when the publisher wrote him a cheque for one million dollars. I covered my scream with my hands, and I just kept saying "That's a sign for me." I was not excited about the money, I felt the man's happiness over his accomplishment when he finished his book. I wanted that same excitement; I needed that same fulfillment. I wanted Luca to exist through words on a page.

Dina paused the show again and sat facing me smiling, "See God is telling you something" she said. I became excited and I told her, "This is what I needed, D can you believe it?" "Yes I believe it" She replied, I started speaking quickly, my face became red, but I could not stop. Dina sat next to me, encouraging me to speak. I went on and on about negative people I had encountered and how I need to let go of the past. I told her I needed to remove myself from nasty and mean people and that I had made the right decision about my baby.

I spoke a mile a minute and I could hardly contain myself. I said, "Maybe God had no plans for me to have a fourth baby and maybe Luca was never meant to be born, but was sent to save me." I knew now this all happened because my life was becoming full of sadness and despair for no apparent reason, without me really realizing it. My ears began to ring and my head felt really tight, as though someone was pushing the sides of my head in as hard as they could. I choked on my words and my throat closed up. Dina brought me a bottle of water and asked, "Are you okay? You sound like you're choking." I drank the water and said, "I feel like my throat is closing and my ears are ringing" but I could not stop talking, "I feel as though I aborted all the pain and all the sadness from the past, I want to move on Dina, I'm ready to move on."

Dina hugged me, "People wait all their lives for an epiphany like this, and you had one." She continued, "My heart feels so happy for you." We finished watching the rest of the show. I did not grasp another word after that, my mind was full and I felt as though all the demons had left my body. I left her house and ran across the street. There was nothing left for me to conquer and I needed to rest.

Angelo was watching television when I walked into the family room. "I saw Dina's car at home. What were you guys doing?" he asked. "Ang, we watched this DVD called The Secret." I tried to explain a bit about it but I could see he was not interested. He began to laugh, "Good, order lots of money from the universe." I felt alone and replied, "I will, you'll see, positive thinking will get us through the hard times." Angelo sat up, "What about your writing? Has that all been forgotten?" "No, I just need some time." I walked away. I did not want Angelo to put down my new thoughts. It was easy enough to do so on my own.

For the next few days I felt happy and I made time to meditate in the evenings. I enjoyed taking baths and the steam from the hot water flowed in the air, making my face sweaty. I loved turning off the lights and lighting candles around the tub. I stared at the fire and the colors fighting their way through. I enjoyed imagining the Angels flying through the flames to visit. I closed my eyes and asked the Angels to gather around me and dance.

Then I thanked them for all the good in my life and asked for guidance in the negative that continuously tried to enter my mind. Most of all, I thanked them for helping me keep my children safe. I also thanked them for being my eyes and ears for Luca.

- 29 -
Mass

One Sunday morning I woke up to the sunny and bright light peering through my bedroom window. I felt happy and wanted to do something special. I needed to go to church, I needed to visit God. I always found mass to be extremely boring and it took great effort not to find excuses to not go. That day seemed different, and I was happy to get dressed, quickly have an espresso, and get out the door. "Does anyone want to come to church?" I asked the children. "No." There was no hesitation on their part, and I giggled. I did not try to convince them to come. For some reason I wanted to go alone, I needed to go alone, I just did not know why.

Regular mass began, and as the priest started the sermon my eyes focused on Jesus hanging on the cross. I could not stop staring at his face and I no longer heard the priest nor felt my surroundings. I just stared at Jesus' face and I could almost see him looking back at me. Tears began to flow down my cheeks and goose bumps trickled up and down my back. Words formed in my mind and I started speaking to Jesus. "I never really looked at your face, oh Lord, and I can't believe how beautiful you really are."

I realized I had never really got to know my faith. My entire life I had studied the words I was taught in the catholic schools and all the years at church, the priests told us what was acceptable. My parents preached all the time, but I never bothered to understand them, all I did was memorize the words. I realized now, that God and the Angels really were listening to me and I truly believed with all my heart that there was something big and magical in the universe, and that they want good for everyone. Most of all, I realized that I was not really living life with my soul; I was living the life of a robot. I followed the rules of my family, I followed the law, I obeyed the traditions of marriage, having children and trying to be the perfect housewife.

- 30 -
Coming Home

I was excited to drive home and be with my family. I knew I would walk in the door and Angelo would be on the sofa watching television while my children played happily with their toys. I tried to catch the green lights so that I would get there as fast as I could. I ran up the driveway and opened the front door, knowing Lucy would try to outrun the boys to be the first to give me a hug. I sat on the floor with a big smile on my face as the children spoke from the top of their lungs trying to over power each other. I laughed as I tried to keep up with "Lucy did this, and Gaetano said that, and Joseph dropped….." "Okay guys, let's start our day with a big breakfast. Go play and I'll call you when it's ready." The children scattered into the playroom. Angelo came into the hallway and extended his hand out to help me up. We embraced each other and I took in a deep breath of his scent. I felt warm and content as my head lay on his chest. Angelo giggled, "I only came over to ask if you were thinking of omelets or scrambled, but hugs are good too." I stared into his gorgeous hazel eyes "Whatever you want baby." I replied.

Angelo followed me into the kitchen and searched for the sausages in the freezer. I watched him move the frozen vegetable out of his way and yet he still struggled to find it. I reached passed him and grabbed the sausages from the shelf. "How do you do that? How do you know where everything is?" Angelo was annoyed. "Ang, why don't you go play with the children and I'll prepare the meal." I said as I nudged him out of the way and closed the freezer door. I watched him walk away as I thought, "I hope you have made peace with yourself. I hope it's not all bottled up inside."

The sausages began to crackle in the pan, I gently turned each one over, and I felt alive. Finding myself brought me back into a body that pumps blood into my veins, a heart that beats to a happy rhythm, and a soul that has awaken from a deep sleep.

I noticed little changes happening to me and I was happy and light. I called everyone to the table and watched the children fight over how many sausages they would get. Angelo buttered the toast and placed a slice on each plate. I poured the orange juice in each glass And placed it next to each plate. "What do you want to do with the kids today?" Angelo asked. "Let's just go to the park and be together. I can bring espresso in a thermos and we can let the kids play." Joseph looked up at me and said, "Sounds like a plan." Angelo and I began to laugh. "Good." I answered. I could not stop staring at my children. I discovered that my children were really little people who are funny and kind. They enjoy running around the house, laughing, and screaming and now I really appreciated those sounds. Everyone hurried to clear the table so we could get on with our day.

I knew the children were already getting their shoes and jackets on, and were anxious to get to the park. I was standing over the sink washing dishes as quickly as I could to join my family. Today was a good day. I thought, "When we get back from the park I will need to take some time to pay a few bills." Then my thoughts went to, "What should I cook for dinner?" My soul felt replenished and I smiled as I thought, "I think tonight our bed time story will have Jacomino and Pasqualino going to the park with their sister Laduica." I thought of all the different adventures our imaginary siblings would go threw when I felt a tug. "When can we go?" Gaetano asked. "I'll be ready in two minutes baby. Just give me two minutes." I watched him walk away as I took a deep breath and thought, "Maybe next week I can convince Angelo to take me to the cemetery to see Luca, but for now it's just another normal day. Thank God, just a normal day."

- 31 -
Final Thoughts

I no longer screamed at my children to find something quiet to do during the day, and I no longer considered only myself. I had not heard the words "Poor Antoinette" in a long time and, frankly, I was tired and weary of always being the focus of attention in my family.

My husband really is my lover and my favorite best friend, together we now appreciated the sky being so blue and if I closed my eyes I could hear the littlest sounds that I took for granted every day.

Life got better and although I still offered my worries to God and the Angels, I also asked Angelo's guardian Angel to guide him through his worries. We still worried about our financial situation but I was thankful that we could still buy food and had a roof over our heads.

As for our decisions, I no longer worried about those who expressed their opinions. I understood they had their own issues that were not for me to deal with. I spent so much time hating them that it took my thoughts away from my sadness, so I thank them in my prayers for helping me through my grieving process.

I sat down at the dining room table and tried to figure out how many minutes I had lived in 42 years. I laughed out loud when I realized that the saddest times in my life were only a small number of minutes in my lifetime. God really loves me if most of the minutes in my life were good. I now understood that it is my choice to be happy and healthy. The universe provided as long as I was specific in my orders and believed.

I do believe that God doesn't give us anything we can't handle. I know now everything that happened was all for a reason that only God will ever know. I do believe with all my heart that my story needed to fall in the hands of someone who needs me. If that person is you, I hope you can find your own peace. May God bless.

- 32 -
Heaven.

I always worried about death. I was never afraid of dying, but I was always afraid of judgment day. I often pictured Saint Peter standing at the pearly white gates asking the big question, "Why do you feel you deserve to enter the gates of heaven?" I could never come up with the right answer. I no longer dwell on my fears. Just as Mother Mary stands next to her son, I have earned the right to stand next to mine. I know our half hearts will, one day, be put together and I know God would not want anything less for his children.

Luca, our time apart just makes us stronger. I am not in a rush to be with you right now, because I know you are safer and happier than anyone on this earth. When my work here is done I will come to you.

Acknowledgements

Thank you God for sending such wonderful people into my life that have loved and supported my family through the good times and the bad.

A special thank you to Angelo, I am grateful for your kindness, your happiness, and, most of all, your love. I love you very much and I thank you for all of your support.

Joseph, Gaetano and Lucy – mommy loves you very much and I hope you always have love, health, and happiness in your lives. You already have special Angels in your lives, embrace them.